MATLAB® Primer for Speech-Language Pathology and Audiology

MATLAB® Primer for Speech-Language Pathology and Audiology

Frank R. Boutsen, PhD, CCC-SLP
Justin D. Dvorak, MS

PLURAL PUBLISHING
INC.

PLURAL PUBLISHING
INC.

5521 Ruffin Road
San Diego, CA 92123

e-mail: info@pluralpublishing.com
Website: http://www.pluralpublishing.com

Typeset in 11/14 Garamond by Flanagan's Publishing Services, Inc.
Printed in the United States of America by McNaughton & Gunn, Inc.

NOTICE TO THE READER
MATLAB® is a registered trademark of The MathWorks, Inc. The use of MATLAB® software does not represent endorsement by MathWorks. MathWorks does not guarantee the accuracy of this publication.

For MATLAB® product information, please contact:
The MathWorks, Inc.
3 Apple Hill Drive
Natick, MA, 01760-2098
USA Tel: 508-647-7000
Fax: 508-647-7001
e-mail: info@mathworks.com
Website: mathworks.com
How to buy: www.mathworks.com/store

Library of Congress Cataloging-in-Publication Data

Boutsen, Frank R., author.
MATLAB primer for speech-language pathology and audiology / Frank R. Boutsen, Justin D. Dvorak.
p. ; cm.
Includes bibliographical references and index.
Includes bibliographical references and index.
ISBN 978-1-59756-653-7 (alk. paper)—ISBN 1-59756-653-5 (alk. paper)
I. Dvorak, Justin D., author. II. Title.
[DNLM: 1. MATLAB. 2. Software. 3. Speech-Language Pathology. 4. Audiology. 5. Computer Simulation. 6. Mathematical Computing. W 26.55.S6]
RC423
616.85'500285—dc23

2015029453

Contents

Foreword

MATLAB is one of the most useful and versatile computational tools available today. It can be used in any field requiring data analysis, prediction, modeling, simulation, or visualization. Unlike software packages that have been written for a specific purpose, MATLAB provides an environment that allows a user to create solutions to quantitative problems. It is truly a *laboratory* stocked with a great set of tools, but to those unfamiliar with computer programming and algorithmic concepts, the point of entry can be rather daunting. This much-needed book opens the door to the laboratory, and guides the user through the basic concepts needed to get started on a path toward creative problem solving. Although intended for students, researchers, and clinicians in Speech Pathology and Audiology, this book is an excellent introduction for anyone wanting to learn to use MATLAB.

As explained in Chapter 1, a particular advantage of MATLAB is that it is an "interpreted" language, which means that when a user types a command or instruction, it is converted to a form that can be used by a computer to deliver an immediate result. Although this seems like the obvious goal of any computer program, it contrasts with using a "compiled" language such as C or C++. For example, one could type "2 + 2" at the MATLAB prompt, press ENTER, and immediately see the answer "4." To get the same result using a compiled language would require writing a short program in a text editor in which a variable, say "*x*," would be declared as a double or single precision number, a line "*x* = 2 + 2" would be written, the file would be saved, and finally it would be submitted to a compiler. Assuming no errors were found and the syntactic rules of the particular language were precisely followed, the compiler would produce an executable version of the program that, when run, would deliver the answer "4." MATLAB effectively shields the user from this back-and-forth process inherent in compiled languages, allowing rapid feedback from command input. This has significant pedagogical advantages that are leveraged in the first chapter as the authors carefully introduce the reader to the computational environment, concepts regarding digital data, and the basic syntax required to represent variables and mathematical expressions. As is the case throughout the book, this chapter includes numerous examples and exercises that encourage the user to interact with MATLAB as the various topics are encountered.

Perhaps the most ubiquitous form of data in Speech Pathology and Audiology is an acoustic signal transduced by a microphone and stored as an audio file. Chapter 2 addresses the relation of sampling frequency and amplitude resolution to acoustic signals, explains the use of specific commands for reading and writing audio files, and demonstrates how to plot signals and play them back for purposes of listening. Other important concepts covered are signal scaling, smoothing, and windowing. Although the main focus of the chapter is on audio signals, commands and functions are also introduced that are applicable to files containing other types of signals such as air flow, fleshpoint motion, electroglottography, and respiration. Of particular importance are the concepts of resampling non-audio signals to coincide with the sampling frequency of an audio signal, thus allowing for multi-signal visualization and analysis.

Another advantage of MATLAB is the relative ease with which it can be integrated with other software packages and used to access a wide range of data file types. For instance, an Excel spreadsheet could be imported into MATLAB where specific columns or rows are assigned to variable names. Some type of processing could then be carried out on these data and, if desired, written back into the original spreadsheet. The examples provided in Chapter 3 demonstrate fairly complex integration of multiple software packages with simple MATLAB scripts that are straightforward to use.

Using concepts presented in the previous chapters, Chapter 4 takes the reader through a range of applications including pure-tone synthesis, formant synthesis, speech in noise, and various forms of signal filtering. Each example is associated with clearly commented blocks of MATLAB code that can be easily implemented. A particularly important aspect of this chapter is the demonstration of how to make use of both built-in MATLAB functions and programs that have been written by other researchers, students, or clinicians.

The final chapter of the book explains how MATLAB can be used to develop code for accessing, managing, and analyzing electronic medical records. Although quite different from the concepts concerning signals, this chapter contains excellent examples of how a system for patient data might be configured, and how those data could be tested and interpreted statistically.

I have been a MATLAB user for about two decades, and utilize it in nearly every aspect of my research and teaching. It has been an ideal environment for developing computational models of speech production, algorithms for processing acoustic, kinematic, and air flow signals, as well as for animating time-varying quantities such as a spectra and vocal tract configurations. I appreciate the difficulties, however, of teaching others to use MATLAB, especially in the absence of a programming background. This book was written to address exactly this niche, and I believe it definitely succeeds in doing so.

—Brad H. Story
Professor and Associate Department Head
Speech, Language, and Hearing Sciences
University of Arizona
Tucson, Arizona

Introduction

About the Text

This book is intended for students, researchers, and clinicians in speech-language pathology and audiology who wish to increase their productivity by incorporating and automating common research procedures and data-analysis calculations, or to develop new tools and methods for their own paradigms and data processing. It assumes no prior knowledge of programming, but requires the reader have a grasp of basic computer skills such as managing folders, moving files, and navigating file paths and folder structures.

It is assumed that the reader is familiar with high-school–level mathematics such as trigonometry, matrix algebra, complex and imaginary numbers, and some calculus (mainly for theoretical understanding of some signal-processing principles). Important points to review are contained in Appendixes A (Review of Trigonometry), B (Review of Complex Numbers), and C (Review of Matrices).

Readers should have the most current academic or student version of MATLAB installed before beginning the programming exercises and projects, as the practice afforded by the interactive MATLAB environment is critical to mastery of the concepts. Because of the emphasis on speech-signal processing throughout the examples, readers are also advised to purchase the Signal Processing Toolbox, whose functions are used periodically in the text.

Familiarity with audio manipulation and analysis software such as Praat (Boersma & Weenik, 2015) and Audacity (Audacity Team, 2015) is helpful for comparison of features and processes, but this is not strictly required.

MATLAB® in Speech-Language Pathology and Audiology

MATLAB has traditionally been the tool of engineering fields, and its usage in speech and hearing has grown since its initial introduction by way of the spatial temporal index, developed by Smith et al. (1995). In the intervening decades, many top laboratories have adopted MATLAB to perform their computationally intensive signal-processing tasks, even developing custom routines and toolboxes to be shared with the research community. Examples include COLEA (Loizou, 1999), the VOICEBOX Speech Processing Toolbox (Brookes, 2013), and the EMATOOLS (Nguyen, 2000) package for analyzing speech and articulation data, among many others. These toolboxes can be used alongside or in addition to MathWorks' own Signal Processing Toolbox (MathWorks, 2015), an add-on product for MATLAB that facilitates spectrogram creation, filter design, and other useful functions for speech analysis.

The philosophy behind this text is that adoption of the type of quantitative mindset useful for MATLAB programming need not conflict with the speech and hearing researcher's or clinician's adaptability. We hope to demonstrate that MATLAB can be integrated seamlessly in the clinic and the laboratory for the purposes of basic research and supplementing evidence-based practice.

Conventions Used

Text in mono-spaced font (e.g., `myVar = rand()`) refers to commands that are to be typed into the MATLAB Command Window, code to be saved in a script, file names, or MATLAB output (indicated with a gray background). When the prompt (>>) is present, this indicates that everything after it is to be typed into the Command Window, and the ENTER key is to be pressed after each line. The interactive engagement with programming material in this way is much more informative than simply reading the book, and students are encouraged to have an active MATLAB session open while reading so they can try out various techniques and commands.

Bolded words are important terms in the programming field that may be unfamiliar to the casual computer user—these will be explained on their first use and will also appear in the Glossary.

Software Resources

In addition to the above named applications, readers may find Notepad++ (a free ASCII text-editor, *not* word-processor) and XVI32 (a free hex editor) useful in examining the example data files provided. XVI32 will be of particular utility in understanding the structure of delimited ASCII files for storing numeric data.

Layout of the Book

Chapter 1 introduces the MATLAB programming environment and offers reasons why speech-language pathologists and audiologists might employ

MATLAB as the platform of choice in research and clinical settings, rather than alternative programming languages such as C++, Visual Basic, or Java. In addition, the reader is informed about computer basics including digital conversion, operations, matrices, functions, and control flow. Readers are prepared to convert analog data to a digital format and to conduct some basic operations. In addition, they are taught how to label, store, and retrieve the data or subsets thereof.

Chapter 2 expands on topics introduced in Chapter 1, with a focus on application to elementary sound acoustics. The implications of discrete-time sampling and limited precision are discussed. In addition, MATLAB code for reading and writing audio files is demonstrated. Manipulation of audio signals through simple matrix operations is explored. At this stage the reader has been prepared for elementary operations on sound objects that set the stage for more detailed and or combined applications, as are needed for building and manipulation of stimuli for clinical and research applications. This chapter lays the groundwork for skills that are addressed in Chapter 4.

Chapter 3 prepares the reader for applications that require integration of an application into a project's workflow. To that end, we discuss options to interface MATLAB to various software tools and programming languages. They include use of direct interface methods (such as prewritten packages) as well as interprocess communication via sockets and temporary files. This chapter provides prerequisite information for Chapter 5.

Chapter 4 builds on skills introduced in Chapter 2, surveying a selection of practical applications of MATLAB programming techniques in both speech-language pathology and audiology. These techniques are applicable anywhere in the continuum from "bench" lab research to live deployment in a clinical setting, and cover generation of stimuli and test items, data collection and analysis, and data management. Combined, these techniques facilitate a wide range of research and clinical activities. Because future applications and software needs are unpredictable, the chapter exercises often go beyond the material in the text, encouraging the reader to discover new functionality and achieve a degree of independence in planning and completing projects.

Chapter 5 continues the discussion initiated in Chapter 3, but now widens the scope to the area of health informatics in the speech and audiology clinic. The discussion focuses on analysis and management of clinic data. Data mining and subsequent knowledge discovery from electronic medical records are addressed. Specifically, patient data are mined to evaluate efficacy and cost effectiveness for the purpose of clinical decision making. The chapter concludes with examples of analyses in a hypothetical, clinical scenario which uses MATLAB as a unifying framework.

Within a chapter, each section includes a variety of student exercises. In general, the earlier exercises test the theoretical knowledge behind a principle, or the proper understanding of terminology used in the fields of programming and signal processing. These are followed by exercises that focus on programming problems, requiring the performance of simple tasks or writing short samples of code (usually less than 10–20 lines) which apply foundational principles and demonstrate correct programming techniques. The final exercises within each section are larger and more complex than programming problems, will often involve novel combinations of principles explained in the text and skills tested in the concepts and programming problems, and are meant to simulate real-world conditions. The gradation of skill level is intended to encourage the reader to seek out or create MATLAB functions beyond those presented in the text, leading to independent programming ability.

Website Support

The authors are aware that it is impossible to cover, within an introductory volume, the wide range of solutions that have been developed in MATLAB for the fields of speech-language pathology and audiology. We anticipate that readers may need additional support and/or information, especially as new problems are discovered and the associated algorithms are implemented. This is especially true in health informatics, which is a rapidly expanding field.

To that end, the textbook website, located at http://www.pluralpublishing.com/publication/mpslpa, is intended to serve as an ever-expanding repository of useful MATLAB functions, exemplary data sets, and solution guides that go beyond the material in the text. The website also includes key code examples from the textbook for easy copying and pasting into the MATLAB editor.

References

Audacity Team. (2015). Audacity [Computer program]. Version 2.1.0. Retrieved from http://web.audacityteam.org/

Boersma, P., & Weenink, D. (2015). Praat: doing phonetics by computer [Computer program]. Version 5.4.09. Retrieved from http://www.praat.org/

Brookes, M. (2013). VOICEBOX: speech processing toolbox for MATLAB [Computer software]. Version 2803. Retrieved from http://www.ee.ic.ac.uk/hp/staff/dmb/voicebox/voicebox.html

Loizou, P. (1999). COLEA: A MATLAB software tool for speech analysis [Computer software]. Retrieved from http://ecs.utdallas.edu/loizou/speech/colea.htm

MathWorks. (2015). Signal processing toolbox [Computer software]. Version R2015a. Retrieved from http://www.mathworks.com/products/signal/

Nguyen, N. (2000). A MATLAB toolbox for the analysis of articulatory data in the production of speech. *Behavior Research Methods, Instruments, and Computers, 32*(3), 464–467.

Smith, A., Goffman, L., Zelaznik, H. N., Ying, G., & McGillem, C. (1995). Spatiotemporal stability and patterning of speech movement sequences. *Experimental Brain Research*, *104*(3), 493–501.

Acknowledgments

I wish to thank those who have contributed in ways large and small, directly and indirectly, and knowingly or not, to the conception and writing of this book. They include my family, my wife, my mentors, and my coauthor. I also wish to thank Dr. Brad Story for kindly agreeing to write the foreword to this book. The idea for this book certainly took hold at many scientific conferences. However, it was my working with MATLAB in the Motor Speech and Prosody Laboratory at the University of Oklahoma Health Sciences Center, as well as the generous support I received from the MathWorks Book Program, that ultimately made it possible to share in this book solutions that readers can learn, modify, and improve as they go about conducting their research and practice in Speech-Language Pathology and Audiology. Lastly, I also would like to extend my gratitude to BIOPAC Systems, Inc. for their generous support.

—FRB

I would like to express my gratitude to my family and friends for their support throughout the writing and publication process. I would also like to thank my students, laboratory colleagues, and research mentor for their many insightful comments and suggestions. Finally, this project could not have been completed without the generous support of the MathWorks Book Program.

—JDD

To our students.

1

Introduction to Programming With MATLAB®

Introduction to MATLAB®

What Is MATLAB®?

MATLAB (short for Matrix Laboratory) is both a programming language and computing environment developed by MathWorks, Inc. (Natick, Massachusetts), and is designed for performing calculations and data processing. It is traditionally used in engineering and other computationally intensive fields due to its ability to handle large data sets and matrices natively. Evidence-based practice, improved tools for speech and language recording, as well as a widening scope of parameters assessed in speech-language pathology practice have changed the assessment in speech pathology from subjective and general to objective and detailed. A host of quantitative measures detailing respiratory and vocal tract functions for speech as well as the neurophysiology of language and reading are now used on a regular basis in speech-pathology practice. Most of these parameters are computationally intensive and therefore a challenge to processing, and keeping them together in a record presents an even greater obstacle. In this book, we will cover the use of MATLAB not only for data processing but also for record keeping relevant to speech-language pathology and audiology.

Of note are several free alternatives to MATLAB, specifically GNU Octave and SciPy (an extension to the Python programming language). With some exceptions, code written for MATLAB is generally compatible with the Octave system, and vice versa. However, for the sake of simplicity, this book adheres to standard MATLAB syntax and assumes the presence of a MATLAB installation.

Why Use MATLAB®?

There are two main reasons why MATLAB is the work environment of choice for speech-language pathologists and audiologists: its intrinsic qualities and its pedagogical advantages. The latter consideration is important as we acknowledge programming skills do not yet figure centrally in either speech-language pathology and audiology training or practice.

MATLAB has a number of desirable features for computational work in speech-language and hearing research. It can natively handle the `.wav` format commonly used in recorded speech, and allows direct operations on audio and other waveform data, such as frequency analysis, amplitude correction, root-mean-square (RMS) calculation, and many others. It can also import large data sets in `.txt`, `.xls`, `.xlsx`, and other common data-storage formats without requiring the user to resort to the low-level file operations (e.g., manually opening and closing files, or dealing with reading binary data byte by byte) common in other languages. Furthermore, many expansion kits known as Toolboxes are available from MathWorks or are freely downloadable online, which allow the user to add functionality to the language as projects or research dictate. Of particular value is the Signal Processing Toolbox, which is capable of online computation, can produce spectrograms and other graphical representations of speech quickly and easily, and contains a number of useful functions for speech analysis.

For the purposes of teaching programming to speech-language pathologists and audiologists, the interactive nature of MATLAB is invaluable. Many other programming languages (e.g., C++ or Java) require sometimes-lengthy compile times between writing the code and seeing the result, which can make it difficult for the beginner to try new ideas or understand why a portion of code does not work as planned. MATLAB, however, executes instructions entered in its Command Window with near-immediate feedback, and thus is favorable to iterative development where a project is tested and modified extensively throughout the development cycle. Furthermore, the abstraction of frequently used code is aided by the use of `.m` files. These `.m` files can be called by any other piece of code without specific inclusion directives—they only need to be in the correct folder or search path. This is used to good effect in developing the concepts of functions and abstraction. On a more technical note, creation of variables in MATLAB is as simple as typing an assignment statement (e.g., `myVar = 12.345`). In Java or C++, variables must be explicitly declared and assigned to a particular data type before they can be used; while this practice does lead to more efficient code, it often proves a stumbling block for new programmers, or even experienced developers when prototyping a new project. MATLAB programmers can concentrate on higher-level abstractions and program semantics without bothering with memory management.

Finally, a sizable body of code already exists in MATLAB for many common speech-processing tasks and theoretical models, including the influential Klatt synthesizer (Klatt, 1980) and the DIVA model (Guenther et al., 2006). And because MATLAB works on Windows, Mac OS X, and Linux, most of this code is easily portable across platforms when appropriate conventions are used. This applies to reader-generated code as well, allowing one to, say, write code on a Mac at home and run it successfully on a PC or Linux machine in the lab or clinic the next day. Throughout the text, we will emphasize code portability when discussing use of file names, paths, and file operations.

Some Disadvantages

We would bc rcmiss to overlook MATLAB's relatively low speed for iteration in extremely computationally intensive operations. Because MATLAB is a high-level, interpreted (not compiled) language, it runs much more slowly than languages closer to the machine's native hardware, like C++, unless proper vectorization techniques are applied. The speed issue can be alleviated through the use of `.mex` files, which are compiled code and run many times faster than the corresponding `.m` files, but which can also require translating the MATLAB code into a compiled language and running it through a separate compiler for each machine architecture (32- vs. 64-bit, e.g.). On Windows machines, precompiled DLL files can also be used with the `calllib()` function. The creation of such files, however, is beyond the scope of this introductory textbook.

The MATLAB® Environment

This is the default layout of the MATLAB window. When MATLAB is freshly installed, its main window, or Desktop, will look similar to Figure 1–1.

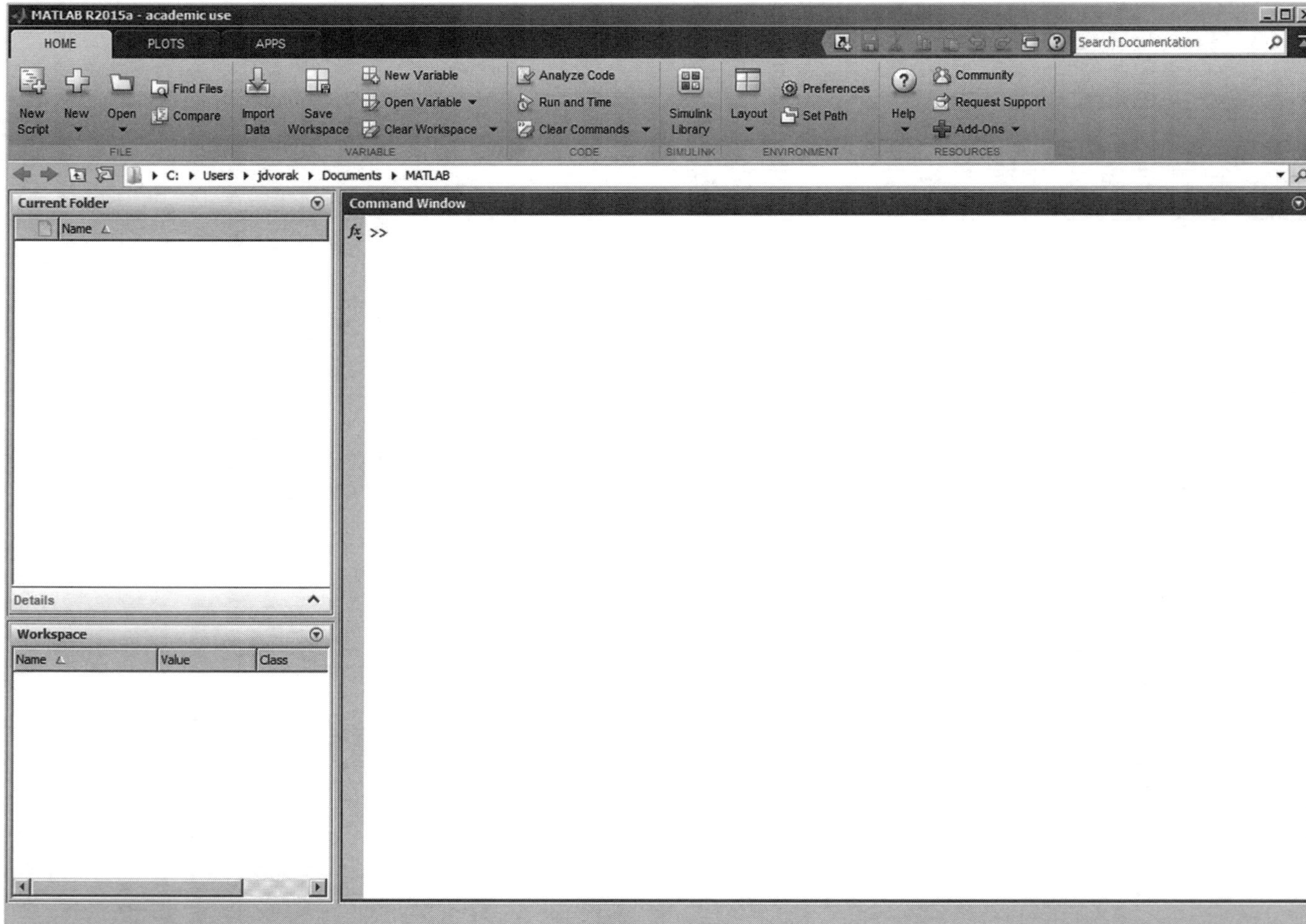

Figure 1–1. Default layout of the MATLAB window.

The topmost element of the Desktop is the Toolstrip, which is a tabbed interface to a wide variety of MATLAB functions and commands. Some functions are specific to the MATLAB environment itself, such as the "New Script" and "Open" buttons, whereas others are more applied, such as those in the "Plots" or "Apps" tabs.

Below the Toolstrip, the desktop is divided into a number of smaller windows, or panels. The most important panel is the Command Window, in which typed commands are executed, calculations are performed, and functions calls are made (Figure 1–2). Commands are entered after the prompt (>>), and submitted by pressing the ENTER or RETURN key. When a calculation is completed, results will also be displayed in the command window unless output is suppressed by terminating the statement with a semicolon (;).

A useful tool for new MATLAB programmers is the Function Browser button, which is indicated as a script *fx* to the left of the prompt in the Command Window. As the name would suggest, clicking on this button allows one to browse through all functions accessible through base MATLAB and any installed Toolboxes, insert them into scripts or the command window, or call up their documentation.

To the left of the Command Window is the Current Folder panel. Organized as a file manager, this panel displays all files and subfolders in the

Figure 1–2. Command window.

current directory. Organization of all data files, scripts, and subfunctions in a single directory allows viewing its contents at a glance without switching from the MATLAB process or disrupting ongoing calculations. The directory shown in the Current Folder panel is also the first place MATLAB will look when making a function call or opening a file. Note that a common beginner's error is to attempt to call a function in another folder without switching to that folder or adding it to the search path.

Below the Current Folder panel is the Workspace, which shows all of the MATLAB variables currently stored in the computer's memory. This is useful for keeping track of intermediate values in a complex procedure or a lengthy set of calculations, as well as for organizing collections of data. Additionally, the contents of the Workspace can be saved and loaded using the `save` and `load` functions, respectively.

The down-arrow icon displayed in the upper-right corner of each panel (Figure 1–3) opens a menu, which allows manipulations such as panel closing, minimization/maximization, or undocking to its own window. Furthermore, depending on the panel, this menu contains additional relevant options. For example, the menu associated with the Workspace allows one to save the Workspace variables to a `.mat` file for later use.

The tool panels can also be resized by dragging their borders, or moved by dragging their titles. Experiment with these tools and rearrange them to suit your needs. Do not worry; if you accidentally close a tool or clutter the layout, all can be restored by clicking the "Layout" button in the "Home" tab, and then selecting "Default."

Even though simple commands can be entered in sequence in the Command Window, most MATLAB programming involves the development of scripts, which are essentially sequences of commands that are executed one after another, and functions, which are custom commands that can be called from the Command Window, from scripts, or even from other functions. Scripts and functions are created in the Editor (Figure 1–4), which is invoked by pressing the "New Script" button.

Figure 1–3. Down-arrow icon.

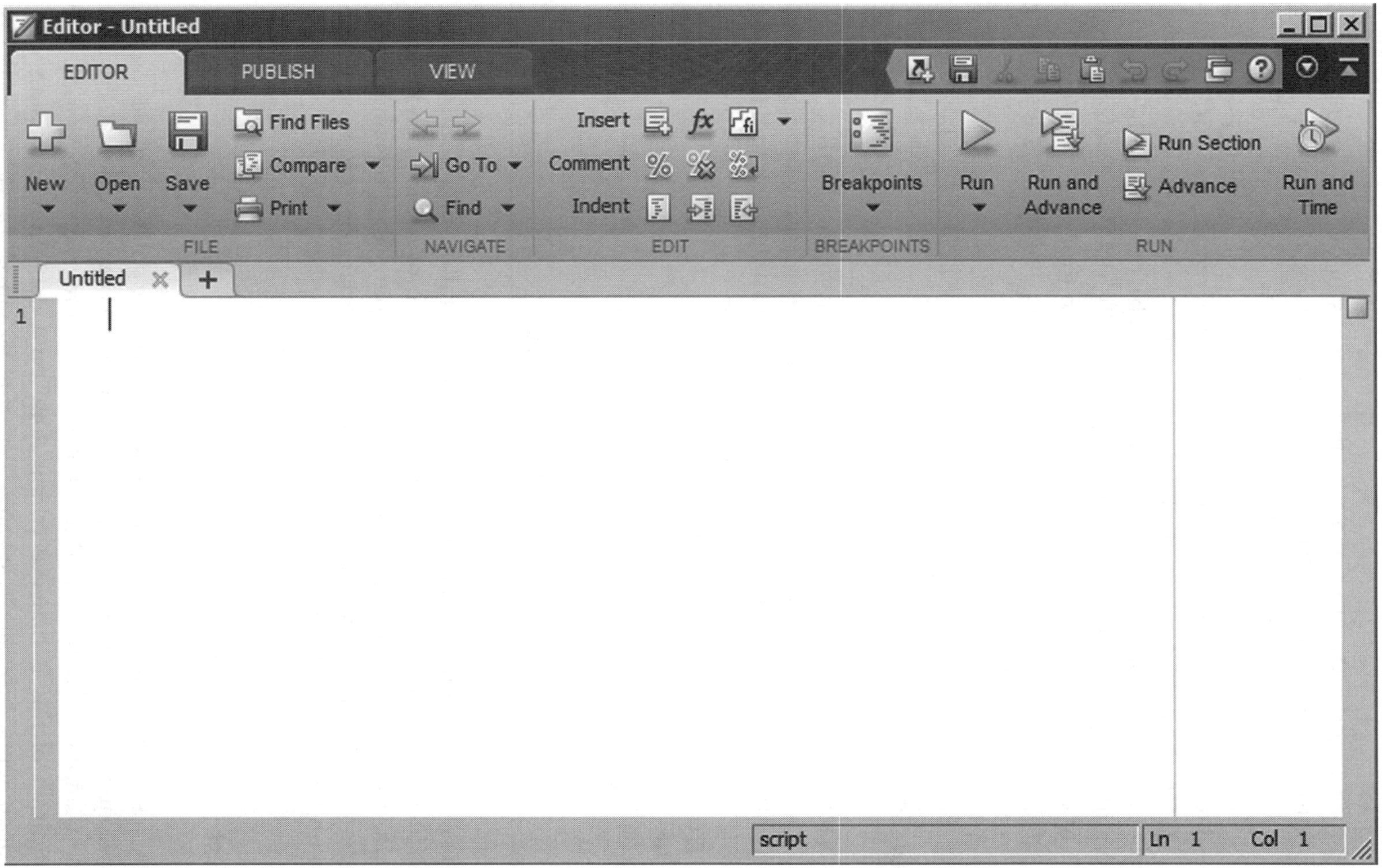

Figure 1–4. Editor window

Much like the Desktop window, the Editor window also organizes its tools into a number of tabs. The "Editor" tab contains tools useful for editing and managing scripts and functions, which are saved as `.m` files. The "Publish" tab is used to insert code markup for MATLAB's built-in publishing capability, which allows the automatic generation of reports and corresponding figures and program outputs. Publishing one's code in this manner is an excellent way to ensure reproducibility in research and can also be used to streamline the generation of clinical reports. Finally, the "View" tab contains tools to customize the arrangement of panes within the Editor window. This is useful when working on a large project involving multiple `.m` files or long sequences of commands.

Exercises

1. Name some advantages and disadvantages of using MATLAB.
2. In your future projects, you will likely need to rearrange the MATLAB Desktop to suit the task at hand. Experiment with the tools and icons on the Desktop. Close each tool and reopen it, arranging it as you see fit. Try maximizing and undocking tools as well.
3. Restore all tools to their default position.

Computer Basics

In this section, fundamental concepts to the operation of a computer are introduced. Topics include computer representation of numeric and textual data, as well as relevant units of information grouping (e.g., bits and bytes). Readers familiar with basic computer science material may skip this section or skim for a brief review.

What Is a Computer?

Many researchers and clinicians use computers every day without asking this simple question. A computer is essentially a very complex calculator with a certain amount of storage and a number of user-interface accessories. The implication of this is that everything done on a computer, including writing documents, browsing websites, listening to music, or viewing photos, involves some form of numerical computation (hence the name), storage, or retrieval. In fact, the book you are reading now was, at one time, stored on a computer as a sequence of numbers representing the characters of the Latin alphabet by a scheme known as ASCII, and myriad calculations were performed to transform these numbers into readable letters of a particular size and shape, whether on the screen or on the printed page. These processes also apply to digital patient records, speech samples, and visual stimuli presented during treatment sessions.

Information Storage

Because modern computer architecture is based on electrical circuits in which current either flows or does not flow, all information is reduced to a series of two states: "on" or "off." These states are represented or coded in the **binary** (base-2) number system as 1 for "on" and 0 for "off." One binary digit is known as a **bit** and can take either of these two values.

Obviously, two values alone are insufficient to express the variety of information we might like to encode in a computer, so groupings of bits in time (e.g., serial data transmission) or space (e.g., memory cells or magnetized regions on a hard drive) are used. Just like in base-10 arithmetic, base-2 relies on positional notation to convey larger values. However, instead of the places signifying powers of 10 (e.g., 1, 10, 100, 1000, etc.), they signify powers of two (1, 2, 4, 8, 16, 32, 64, etc.) (Table 1–1).

Some of these binary values may be familiar as they are often used in measures of computing power (e.g., 32- and 64-bit computers). As an aside, these values have important compatibility consequences for operating systems and applications. Most modern operating systems are designed for a 64-bit address space, which allows a greater amount of RAM to be used, but can lead to incompatibilities with earlier, 32-bit software. MATLAB has

Table 1–1. Selected Binary Values

Binary Number	Place-Value Breakdown	Decimal Value
1	1 × 1	1
10	1×2 + 0×1	2
11	1×2 + 1×1	3
100	1×4 + 0×2 + 0×1	4
...		
1000	1×8	8

support for both 32-bit and 64-bit architectures; however, drivers and pre-compiled `.mex` files are generally incompatible without recompilation, which is beyond the scope of this text.

Bits can be expressed in higher-order groupings. The most common grouping is known as a **byte** and represents 8 bits in order from highest to lowest power of 2. When converted to decimal in this way, a byte can take on any value from 0 (all bits set to 0) to 255 (all bits set to 1). Rather than writing eight binary digits for every byte, however, computer scientists find it convenient to break each byte into two halves, and to encode each half as a single **hexadecimal** (base-16) digit, or "hex" digit, for short. Unlike in base-10 arithmetic, hexadecimal requires the addition of six symbols to represent the values from 10 to 15: A, B, C, D, E, and F. As such, one hexadecimal digit can encode 16 unique values (`0` to `F`), and two hexadecimal digits ($16 \times 16 = 256$) can encode one byte ($2^8 = 256$). Again, positional notation is key: each hexadecimal place represents a power of 16, not 10 (Table 1–2).

In MATLAB, the underlying representation of a simple integer in hexadecimal and binary can be seen through use of the `dec2hex` and `dec2bin` functions. The `dec2hex` function converts a decimal number to its hexadeci-

Table 1–2. Selected Hexidecimal Values With Binary and Decimal Equivalents

Hexadecimal	Binary	Decimal
00	0000 0000	0
01	0000 0001	1
02	0000 0010	2
...	...	...
09	0000 1001	9
0A	0000 1010	10
...	...	...
0F	0000 1111	15
10	0001 0000	16
11	0001 0001	17
...	...	...
1F	0001 1111	31
20	0010 0000	32
...	...	...
FF	1111 1111	255

mal representation, whereas the `dec2bin` function goes further and converts displays the underlying binary representation. Although these functions see little use in speech-language pathology or audiology work, they provide a useful and accessible window into a computer's inner workings.

A subset of possible values taken on by a 1-byte number, namely, the range from 32 to 126, can also be used to represent letters in the Latin alphabet, as we will explore in the next section.

Representation of Text

A straightforward application of the use of numeric code for representing an array of elements is the representation of text in **ASCII** code. ASCII (American Standard Code for Information Interchange) is a 7-bit code used in digital electronic systems such as computers and telecommunications equipment where characters of English text (e.g., "a") are each encoded in 1 byte. Note that spaces and punctuation are also considered characters; therefore, the string `'Hello, world!'` requires 13 bytes to store, even though it only contains 10 graphemes. Even the modern Unicode standard is based in part on the ASCII table, so knowledge thereof is useful for dealing with multilingual text and corpora.

A partial ASCII table is provided in Table 1–3 for your reference. Try opening a text file (`.txt`, **not** `.doc` or `.docx`) in a hex editor (e.g., XVI32) and observe the correspondence between the printed alphabetic characters and the hexadecimal digits. In fact, even "numeric" data in delimited text files use this scheme to encode the digits of each number as text characters.

The character corresponding to the decimal number 32 (`20` in hexadecimal) represents a space and is considered a "printable" character. Values before this point (from 0 to 31, decimal) are control codes and are not printable. Code `7F` (127 in decimal) is not considered a printable character either.

In MATLAB, one can easily see the character corresponding to a given decimal number, or vice versa, through the use of the `char()` and `double()` functions, respectively.

Loading Files

When a program "loads" a data file, data from the computer's hard disk are copied into the computer's **random access memory** or RAM. The data on the hard disk may be fragmented into multiple pieces, and some alteration of the order of bytes in the file may have occurred during this process. Even so, once in RAM any change made to the file is not reflected on the hard drive until the file is saved.

Table 1–3. ASCII: American Standard Code for Information Interchange (Printable Range)

Decimal	Hex	Character	Decimal	Hex	Character	Decimal	Hex	Character
32	20		64	40	@	96	60	`
33	21	!	65	41	A	97	61	a
34	22	"	66	42	B	98	62	b
35	23	#	67	43	C	99	63	c
36	24	$	68	44	D	100	64	d
37	25	%	69	45	E	101	65	e
38	26	&	70	46	F	102	66	f
39	27	'	71	47	G	103	67	g
40	28	(	72	48	H	104	68	h
41	29	)	73	49	I	105	69	i
42	2A	*	74	4A	J	106	6A	j
43	2B	+	75	4B	K	107	6B	k
44	2C	,	76	4C	L	108	6C	l
45	2D	-	77	4D	M	109	6D	m
46	2E	.	78	4E	N	110	6E	n
47	2F	/	79	4F	O	111	6F	o
48	30	0	80	50	P	112	70	p
49	31	1	81	51	Q	113	71	q
50	32	2	82	52	R	114	72	r
51	33	3	83	53	S	115	73	s
52	34	4	84	54	T	116	74	t
53	35	5	85	55	U	117	75	u
54	36	6	86	56	V	118	76	v
55	37	7	87	57	W	119	77	w
56	38	8	88	58	X	120	78	x
57	39	9	89	59	Y	121	79	y
58	3A	:	90	5A	Z	122	7A	z
59	3B	;	91	5B	[	123	7B	{
60	3C	<	92	5C	\	124	7C	|
61	3D	=	93	5D	]	125	7D	}
62	3E	>	94	5E	^	126	7E	~
63	3F	?	95	5F	_			

Unformatted text files, often indicated by the extensions `.txt` or `.csv`, usually contain data encoded in ASCII. In contrast, binary or proprietary file formats may use alternative tables or coding systems, which may assign their own meanings, functions, or values to each possible byte. Audio (`.wav`) files are examples of this type, as are MATLAB's own `.mat` files. Later in the text we discuss several easy-to-use MATLAB functions for dealing with common binary and proprietary formats, such as Microsoft Excel's `.xls` or `.xlsx`.

Exercises

1. Why must digital computer information ultimately be coded in binary?
2. Convert the hexadecimal value `2A` to decimal and binary.
3. How would the decimal integer 105 be represented in binary?
4. How many bytes at a minimum would be required to hold a value of 355? How many bits?
5. Translate the binary number 01001101 to decimal. Using Table 1–3, what character or letter does this represent?
6. Assume you have an instrument that communicates with your experimental control computer through a custom cable that can only send or receive 6 bits at a time. For your experiment, each stimulus number is transmitted to the instrument as a single positive integer. How many unique stimulus codes could you send over this cable?

Operators and Variables

In this section, the reader is introduced to the use of operators and basic mathematical functions. Furthermore, assignment of values to variables and differences in data types are addressed. Evaluation of expressions is explained through iterative simplification. Thus, it is made apparent how each component of a complex expression can be reduced to its evaluated value and then substituted into other functions or operators.

Expressions

Expressions are the building blocks of MATLAB programming. Simply put, an expression is anything that can be evaluated, or calculated, by the MATLAB environment. Expressions can include

- Numbers, for example, `123`, `5.432`, or even things like `5.31e3` (the `e` here being used to represent scientific notation: 5.31×10^3)

- Variable names
- Function calls
- Mathematical operators and formulae
- Other expressions

MATLAB generally evaluates an expression from the inside out. It does so following simple algebraic rules. For example, the expression `cos((1+2)/3-1)` becomes, in turn,

- `cos(3/3-1)`
- `cos(1-1)`
- `cos(0)`
- `1`

(We will conduct iterative expression evaluation as needed to show how evaluations proceed.)

Operators

As a technical computing platform, MATLAB implements many mathematical **operators**, including the obvious +, −, *, /, and also ^ for exponentiation. Furthermore, MATLAB includes functions such as `sqrt()` and `log10()` to calculate the square root and base-10 logarithm of an **operand (argument)**, respectively. (The numbers taken by an operator or function are referred to as operands or **arguments**, the latter being a common term in programming.) A full suite of trigonometric functions is also available (e.g., `sin()` and `cos()`), and will prove invaluable for later exercises in waveform synthesis and analysis. For symbolic operators such as +, entering in a command is the same as on any simple calculator (e.g., `5 + 7`). For functions, the **argument** goes within the parentheses (e.g., `sqrt(2)`). Try entering the following mathematical computation at the Command Window and observe how MATLAB reports the result:

```
>> 5 * 20

ans =

 100
```

When multiple operators are used in an expression, some are more tightly bound to their arguments than others; that is, their evaluation precedes that of other operators. This hierarchy is addressed in basic algebraic rules as detailed in basic mathematics. To change the order of operations in MATLAB, simply use parentheses for grouping as you would when writing a standard mathematical equation. Note that you must *not* use brackets ([or]) for alternating levels as some mathematical authors do, as these are reserved for construction of arrays and matrices. Try the following computation to get a feel for grouping operators and functions. Mathematically inclined readers may recognize this as a formula for calculating *phi*, otherwise known as the "golden ratio":

```
>> (1 + sqrt(5)) / 2

ans =

    1.6180
```

In general, spaces between operands and operators are not necessary but are included for clarity. On a final note, all symbolic operators are actually human-readable "syntactic sugar" for underlying functions that perform the same operation. For example, the expression `1 + 2` actually calls the built-in function `plus(1, 2)`. Although the syntax varies, the semantics are the same: both expressions involve passing `1` and `2` as arguments to a function which returns their sum.

The reader may have noticed that MATLAB has been returning the result of these computations using something called `ans`, which also appears in the Workspace window. This is an example of a variable, which we will now explore.

Variables

A **variable** is nothing more than a human-readable name for a location or address in the computer's memory where data are stored. This gives programmers a way to keep track of intermediate results and call them back when needed. In speech and language research, variables are most often in the form of integers (e.g., `5`), floating-point numbers (e.g., `5.0152`), strings (e.g., `'five'`), or ordered sequences of numbers (e.g., `[1.618, 2.718, 3.142]`)—this latter form is explored in far greater detail in **Chapter 3** when dealing with audio data. In almost all cases, a variable name can be used wherever a numeric or string constant can. For example, instead of typing `1+2` in the Command Window, try the following:

```
>> myVar = 1;
>> myVar + 2

ans =

     3
```

Here, MATLAB accepts the data pointed at by the variable `myVar` as an input to the + operator. The second statement is considered an expression, and evaluates as so:

- `myVar + 2`
- `1 + 2` (The value 1 is stored in `myVar`, so the subexpression `myVar` evaluates to 1.)
- `3`

Naming Variables

Variables must be named according to certain conventions. Violating these will result in a syntax error and a nonfunctional program:

- Variable names must start with an alphabetic character (`a-z` or `A-Z`).
- Variable names may not contain nonalphanumeric characters (e.g., %, #, etc.), with the exception of the underscore.
- Variable names should be no longer than 63 characters (the default value of `namelengthmax` in the MATLAB environment).
- Characters after the first may be alphanumeric or an underscore (_).
- Variables are case sensitive, so `MyVariable` is not the same entity as `myvariable`. This contrasts with some other programming languages such as SAS or BASIC. MATLAB will generally try to find a match to an incorrectly capitalized variable name, but if the names are only one letter off, your program will not function without modification.
- Variables must not be given the same names as reserved keywords.

There are also some guidelines for naming variables. Adherence to these guidelines will make your program easier to read and may prevent unexpected or unintended operation; however, they are not strictly necessary for a program to execute:

- Use a consistent naming style throughout your project.
- Use one of the following styles:
  - `mixedCaseVariableNames`
  - `variable_names_with_underscores`
- Use descriptive and unique variable names when practical:
  - Do not use, for example, `sl` for "signal length" if you can afford `signal_length`, `signalLength`, or even `sigLen`.
  - Do not name variables after preexisting functions or constants (more on this later).

- Try to avoid using `i` or `j` as counters in loops, as they may mask the built-in reference to the imaginary unit; this could possibly lead to confusing bugs when designing signal-processing algorithms. Instead, use a more descriptive counter name such as `fileNumber`. This will make later understanding of nested loops far easier.
- If multiple units are used (e.g., seconds, milliseconds, samples), consider naming your variables with a unit suffix. For example, if the variable `signal_length` is expressed in seconds, samples, frames, or minutes, preferences should be given to `signal_length_seconds`, `signal_length_samples`, `signal_length_minutes`, and so on. At the time the code is written, units may seem obvious, but they may not be a week or a month later. This is especially helpful when your program requires unit conversion, for example, for graphical display to the user.

Assignment and Initialization

Assignment to variables in MATLAB is simple. Open your installation of MATLAB, and in the Command Window, type the command `a = 5`. You will see a new variable appear in the Workspace named `a`, unsurprisingly with the value of `5`. You will also see immediate feedback under the command you just typed, displaying the result of the computation—that is, `5`, as follows:

```
>> a = 5

a =

     5
```

Any variable can be used as an operand, or argument, of any of the operators discussed above. For example, try entering the following two lines in your Command Window (note that the `;` is used to suppress output from the first command, but the assignment still takes place):

```
>> b = 2;
>> sqrt(b)

ans =

    1.4142
```

In addition, your Workspace should now show three variables, `a`, `ans`, and `b`. `ans` is a special MATLAB variable designed to contain the result of the most recently performed calculation, and in this case contains the numerical value calculated from the expression `sqrt(b)`. It is therefore ill advised to use `ans` as a variable name, as its contents are liable to be overwritten without warning and may result in incorrect calculations.

Typing `clear` followed by the name of the variable you wish to be removed clears that variable from the workspace. This is usually done when starting a new task or to free up resources by deleting a large matrix or data set. Typing `clear all` removes all of the variables. Try clearing all of the variables now. After doing so, you should notice that the Workspace has become empty.

A variable must be initialized, or filled with some value, before being used. If you repeat the command `sqrt(b)` that you typed in before clearing the variable `b`, MATLAB will generate an error, because the name `b` is no longer meaningful after it has been cleared.

Predefined Constants and Masking

MATLAB includes a number of useful constants as predefined variables or functions, such as `i`, `pi`, and others. As these constants are built into the language, they do not show up in the Workspace. Note that it is possible to create a variable by the same name and accidentally **mask** the default value of the constant, for example, if you type `pi = 3`, all future references to `pi` will evaluate to `3` instead of the correct value. Should this happen, simply clear the variable in error, and the default constant value will be properly referenced the next time the name is used.

Masking can also affect called functions if assigned names are the same as that of a built-in or user-defined function. To avoid this, use descriptive and unique variable names (e.g., prefer `signal_length` or `length_seconds` to just `length`, which is actually a built-in function to determine the length or longest dimension of a matrix or vector).

A useful technique to avoid accidentally masking a predefined constant or function is to type the prospective variable name in the Command Prompt for evaluation. To see this in action, clear all variables from the workspace and type the following:

```
>> length
Error using length
Not enough input arguments.
```

This error message indicates that length is already defined as a function that expects some input arguments. If, however, a unique variable name is entered at the prompt before being initialized, the following will occur, informing you that using this name will not mask any other constants, variables, or functions. In this one case, the error message is actually good news:

```
>> my_unique_name
Undefined function or variable 'my_unique_name'.
```

This error message tells you that the name is not currently known to MATLAB, and is therefore available for assignment without worrying about masking.

Classes of Variables

When a variable is **initialized**, it also gains a class. This tells the MATLAB interpreter what kind of data are referenced by the name. The two most basic variable types for speech and language processing work are doubles (short for double precision floating-point) and characters.

Doubles

In speech science (specifically, in digitized recordings of speech), doubles most often represent what are commonly referred to as "decimal" numbers (i.e., non-whole numbers, or real numbers). For example, if you enter `a = 1.23` in the Command Window, `a` will be considered a variable of class "double." Such variables can serve as arguments to any standard mathematical operator or function. These contrast with integers, which represent whole numbers only. In theory, a real-valued variable can take on an infinite range of values between any two points on the number line, but this is limited in practice by the precision with which the variable is stored.

It is useful to know that a double will take 8 bytes of RAM, although its underlying bit-by-bit representation (IEEE Standard 754) is beyond the scope of this text. When dealing with high-precision data, it is important to understand that some round-off error can occur when dealing with data that differ by extremely small values. The precision of your system can be informally measured by calling the `eps()` function, which returns the smallest possible distance between two doubles (usually equal to 2^{-52} or approximately 2.22×10^{-16}. Fortunately, speech recordings rarely require such precision.

Characters

As outlined above, characters are used to store textual data, and strings are simply arrays of characters. In MATLAB, character-type variables are created by assigning a string of some length (possibly zero) to a valid variable name. Strings are indicated with single quotes, as in the string `'MATLAB'`. For example, the following command creates a variable containing the string `'MATLAB'`:

```
>> lang = 'MATLAB';
```

Using the `double()` function as outlined above, one can easily pass in a string to determine the corresponding ASCII codes of each of its characters:

```
>> double('This is a test string with spaces and punctuation.')
```

Exercises

1. Name the two basic variable classes discussed in this chapter and how they might be useful for speech and language research.
2. A programmer wants to store some "scratch" values in the variables `h`, `i`, `j`, `k`, `l`. What are two reasons why this might be inadvisable?
3. In analyzing a signal and searching for a region of interest, a programmer stores the time points in two variables (`begin` and `end`) to demarcate the region. What is wrong with this approach? Hint: Try entering both proposed variable names into the Command Prompt and observe the results.
4. Create two strings, one for your first name and one for your last name. Using those two strings only, calculate the total length of your name, including the space between your first and last name. Hint: Use the `length()` function.
5. The Caesar cipher is a simple cryptographic algorithm in which each character is shifted up by three in the character ordering (e.g., 'A' becomes 'D') and wrapping around at the end (e.g., 'Z' becomes 'C'). Create a scaled-down version of the Caesar cipher that can encode a single string. For now, ignore the wrap-around process.

Matrices

Overview

A **matrix** is a two-dimensional array of values. The application of matrices in advanced mathematics is pervasive, ranging from statistical analysis, manipulation of correlated data sets and time-series, and processing of medical imaging data. In speech and language applications, a matrix that is likely to be encountered is the two-channel (stereo) sound sample, saved as a `.wav` file. This matrix generally contains many rows, representing the data at each time sample, and two columns, one for each channel. For an idea of how many rows may be involved in working with even a small sound sample (e.g., 0.75 seconds), multiply a standard sampling rate (e.g., 44100 Hz) by the length in seconds to get

```
>> sample_length = 44100 * 0.75

sample_length =
        33075
```

It would be impractical to show the numerical values of a full `.wav` file in text, so let us generate a simplified version of a `.wav` file by calling the `rand()` function, which returns uniformly random `double` data ranging from 0 to 1. We will create a scaled-down simulation of a `.wav` file with five samples and two channels by calling `rand(5,2)`:

```
>> y = rand(5,2) % Generate random, simplified signal.

y =

    0.8147    0.0975
    0.9058    0.2785
    0.1270    0.5469
    0.9134    0.9575
    0.6324    0.9649
```

Note that the `rand()` function generates values between 0 and 1, but the `.wav` specification allows values to range from −1 to 1. Multiplying our simulated signal by 2 and subtracting 1 will cause all results to lie in this range. Notice how a matrix `M` can be multiplied by a scalar `c` by placing the scalar **before** the * sign (`M = c * M`):

```
>> y = 2 * rand(5,2) - 1 % Scale values to resemble a .wav file.

y =

   -0.6848   -0.7162
    0.9412   -0.1565
    0.9143    0.8315
   -0.0292    0.5844
    0.6006    0.9190
```

We can plot the data generated by calling the highly useful `plot()` function with the simulated data as its argument (Figure 1–5):

```
% Plot all columns of the simulated signal.
plot(y)

% Label X and Y axes.
xlabel('Time (samples)')
ylabel('Amplitude')

% Give the plot a title.
title('Simulated Data')
```

Notice the two different lines used to draw each channel. By default, blue (darker line) is used for the first column of matrix data, and orange (lighter line) for the second. Other default colors are used for further columns, but these can all be changed as desired.

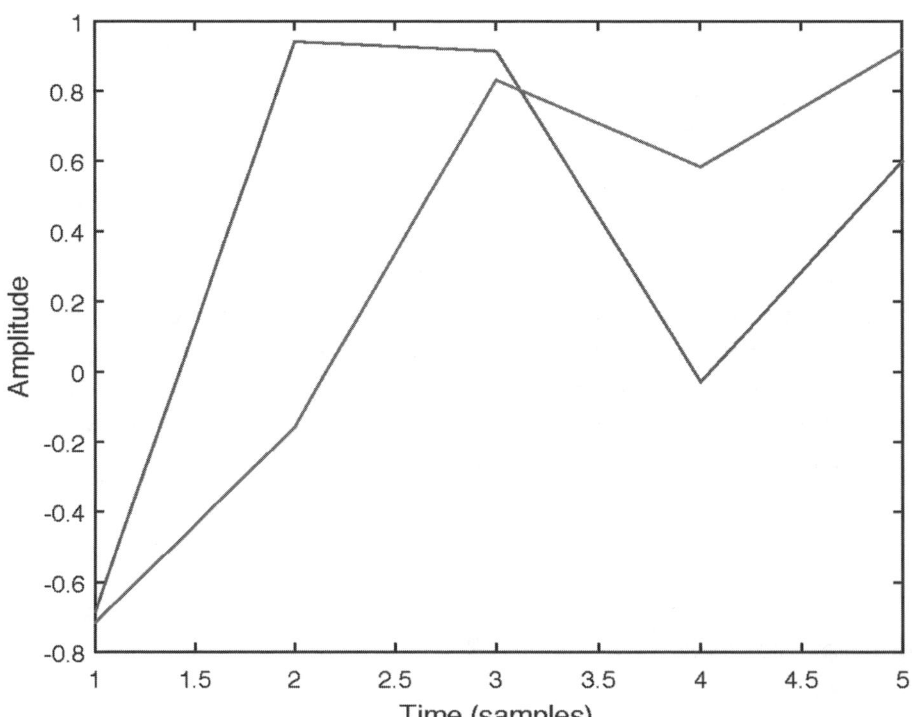

Figure 1–5. Simulated data.

Informative Operations

We now explore some common matrix operations with this data set. For working with audio, one of the most common procedures is to calculate the length of the signal before performing further operations. This can be done by passing the matrix holding the signal as an argument to the `length()` function:

```
>> length(y)

ans =

  5
```

This takes the length of the longest dimension of the matrix, which in audio data will almost always be the number of rows. Keep in mind that the unit of measurement for this result is **samples**. To find the length of the signal in seconds, it is necessary to divide by the sampling frequency used. For example, if our sample "wave" were read in using `[y, fs] = audioread('sample.wav')` and `fs` were set to 44100, then the following calculation would give the length in milliseconds:

```
>> length_ms = length(y) / fs * 1000

length_ms =

    0.1134
```

The `size()` function returns more detailed information than `length()`. Specifically, for a matrix with *r* rows and *c* columns, `size(M)` will return the matrix `[r, c]`:

```
>> size(y)

ans =

     5     2
```

This will prove highly useful for checking the orientation of a signal matrix before proceeding to perform further operations.

Flips

For simple modifications, the `fliplr()` and `flipud()` functions can be used, as may have been guessed, to flip the data in the horizontal and vertical dimensions, respectively. Note that as wave data are stored in columns, a vertical flip (accomplished with `flipud()`) will reverse the audio (i.e., it will play backward) (Figure 1–6), whereas a horizontal flip (`fliplr()`) will reverse the channels (Figure 1–7):

```
>> y_reverse = flipud(y) % Reverse signal.

y_reverse =

    0.6006    0.9190
   -0.0292    0.5844
    0.9143    0.8315
    0.9412   -0.1565
   -0.6848   -0.7162

>> % Plot the reversed signal.
>> plot(y_reverse)
>> xlabel('Time (samples)')
>> ylabel('Amplitude')
>> title('Reversed Signal')

>> % Flip L and R channels.
>> y_channel_flip = fliplr(y)

y_channel_flip =

   -0.7162   -0.6848
   -0.1565    0.9412
    0.8315    0.9143
    0.5844   -0.0292
    0.9190    0.6006

>> % Plot flipped signal.
>> plot(y_channel_flip)
>> xlabel('Time (samples)')
>> ylabel('Amplitude')
>> title('Signal with Flipped Channels')
```

Of particular importance in any work involving matrices is the transpose operation, which switches all rows and columns by effectively rotating the matrix around a 45° axis from the top-left corner. In MATLAB, transposition can be achieved using the postfix `'` operator, as in `M = M'`,

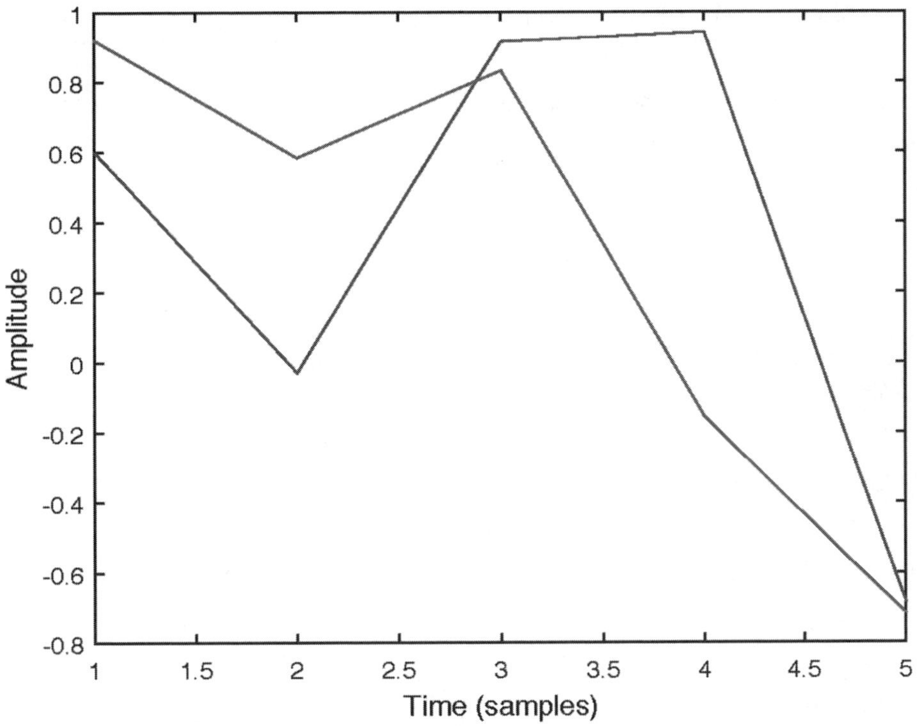

Figure 1–6. Reversed signal.

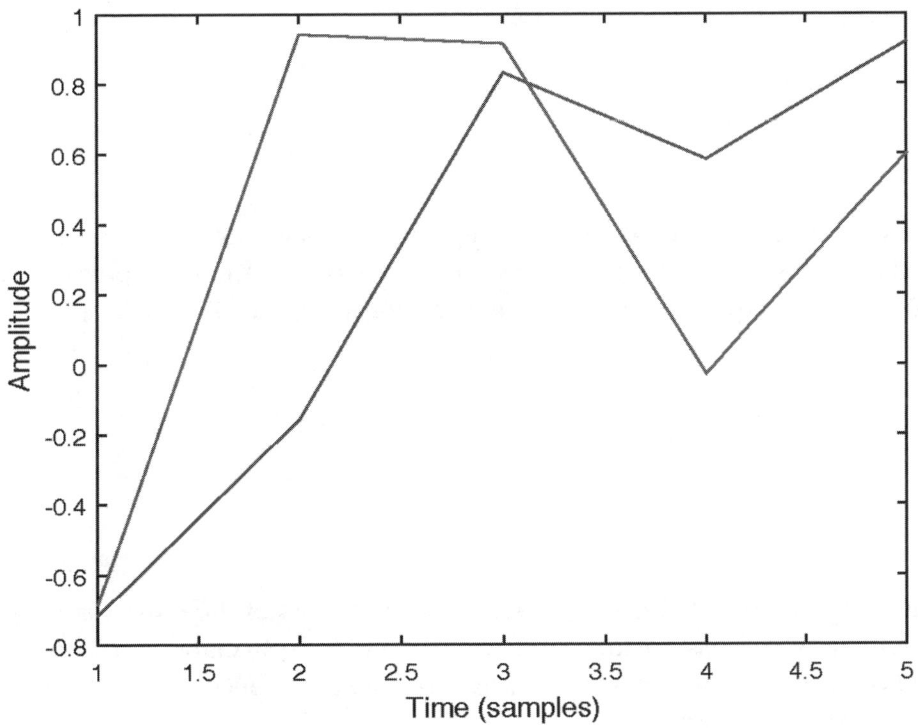

Figure 1–7. Signal with flipped channels.

or the `transpose()` function, as in `M = transpose(M)`. Both notations are equivalent:

```
>> % Create a simple, 3*3 matrix.
>> M = [1 2 3; 4 5 6; 7 8 9]
M =

     1     2     3
     4     5     6
     7     8     9

>> % Use unary transpose operator.
>> M_trans1 = M'

M_trans1 =

     1     4     7
     2     5     8
     3     6     9

>> % Call transpose function.
>> M_trans2 = transpose(M)

M_trans2 =

     1     4     7
     2     5     8
     3     6     9
```

Note that MATLAB does not keep track of the transposition state of a matrix. That is, if our sample matrix were transposed and then plotted, MATLAB would interpret it as a 5-channel, 2-sample signal (Figure 1–8):

```
>> plot(y')
```

Indexing

As it is often critical to be able to access some subset of the entire data signal, we will now discuss various methods of indexing a matrix (selecting elements). Supplying a scalar value *n* as an index will access the *nth* element of the matrix, columnwise:

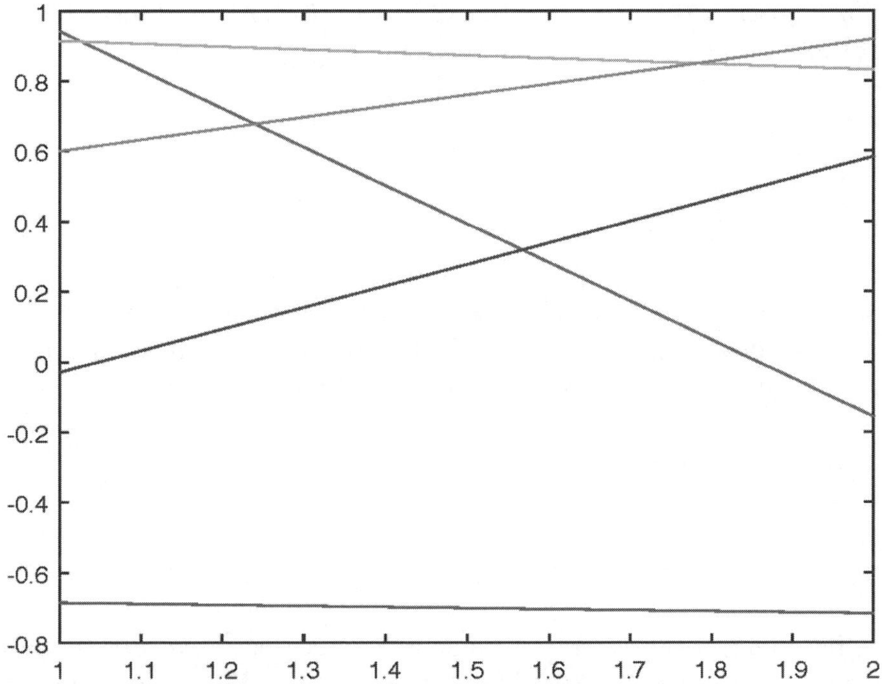

Figure 1–8. Five-channel, two-sample signal.

```
>> y

y =

   -0.6848   -0.7162
    0.9412   -0.1565
    0.9143    0.8315
   -0.0292    0.5844
    0.6006    0.9190

>> first_element = y(1);

first_element =

   -0.6848

>> second_element = y(2);

second_element =

    0.9412
```

If *n* is greater than the number of rows, MATLAB will move on to the next column and resume counting from the top:

```
>> sixth_element = y(6)

sixth_element =

   -0.7162
```

To precisely specify which row and column we want, we can use two-dimensional indexing, as in `M(r,c)`. Selecting the element of our example signal in the first row and second column is done as follows:

```
>> y(1,2)

ans =

   -0.7162
```

Notice that this gives the same result as `y(6)`, because 6 exceeds the number of rows (5), causing MATLAB to "wrap" around to the second column and retrieve the first element therein.

Indexing Errors and How to Prevent Them

Attempting to access an element out of the range of the matrix will result in an error. In most cases, so will attempting to access a fractional index: it makes no sense to look for the 2.5th element of a matrix, for example. In the section on conditionals, we discuss methods to check the size of a matrix and perform adjustments as necessary. However, another approach is to make use of the `max()`, `min()`, `mod()`, and rounding functions. Suppose we wish to access an element *n* of an *r* by *c* matrix *M*, where the variable `n` is the result of some computation which may return a value such that $n <= 0$ or $n > rc$:

```
>> some_value_1 = 3;
>> some_value_2 = 4;
>> n = some_value_1 - some_value_2 % Represents some low-value computation

n =

-1
```

By wrapping this potentially error-inducing `n` in the expression `max(n, 1)`, we can ensure that even if `n` would be too small, the total expression will evaluate to within the bounds of the matrix:

```
>> r = 3;
>> c = 2;
>> M = rand(r,c)

M =

 0.5055 0.9710
 0.3982 0.9051
 0.8259 0.8053

>> low_index = max(n,1)

low_index =

   1

>> M(low_index)

ans =

 0.5055
```

Similarly, even if the value of `n` exceeds *rc*, the expression `min(n, r*c)` will stay within the bounds of the matrix:

```
>> n = some_value_1 * some_value_2 % Represents some high-value computation

n =

 12

>> high_index = min(n, r*c)

high_index =

   6

>> M(high_index)

ans =

 0.8053
```

Suppose instead that `n` is calculated as the sample index corresponding to a supplied time index in milliseconds; that is, for a time `time_ms`, `n = time_ms / 1000 * fs`. This could easily generate fractional values for `n`:

```
>> time_ms = 7;
>> n = time_ms / 1000 * fs

n =

 308.7000
```

Using the `round()` function can help prevent indexing errors:

```
>> M = rand(1000,1);

>> integer_index = round(n)

integer_index =

 309

>> M(integer_index)

ans =

 0.6231
```

Subsetting

The `:` operator can be used in the form `a:b` to create a vector of integers from `a` to `b`, counting by 1:

```
>> elements = 1:4

elements =

  1  2  3  4
```

We can use this operator to create a list of element indices to access in the sample matrix as follows:

```
>> y(1:4,1)

ans =

   -0.6848
    0.9412
    0.9143
   -0.0292
```

This returns Samples 1 through 4 from Channel 1. To access all of the samples in a given channel, however, simply omit the arguments to the : operator:

```
>> y(:,1)

ans =

   -0.6848
    0.9412
    0.9143
   -0.0292
    0.6006
```

Similarly, to access both channels' data for a given sample, use the : operator in the **column** position of the indexing expression:

```
>> desired_sample = 3;
>> y(desired_sample,:)

ans =

    0.9143    0.8315
```

The `end` *Function*

When used in an indexing expression, `end` represents the last index. In our example data, `y(end)` return the last element of `y`, again counting column-wise (the last element in the last column):

```
>> y(end)

ans =

 0.4808
```

To control which column is accessed, simply use both a row and column index, as follows:

```
>> y(end,1)

ans =

    0.6006
```

Exercises

1. A fellow student has imported a two-channel wave file and performed some operations on it. You have received the matrix he was working with for further analysis. Although checking its length with the `length()` function gives you a reasonable value, when you attempt to plot the data, you get a graph full of many short lines, as opposed to two long, detailed signals. What might have happened? Which function could you call to determine this, and what might its output reveal?
2. You have imported a wave file with 12,322,045 samples, which was recorded at 48000 Hz. The signal is saved in the variable `y`, and its sampling frequency in `fs`. In one line of code, calculate the length of this signal in minutes. Evaluations resulting in a fractional minute (e.g., 2.57 minutes) are acceptable.
3. Write one line of code to extract only the left channel from a stereo `.wav` file imported to a matrix `y`.
4. Write one line of code to extract only the right channel from a stereo `.wav` file imported to a matrix `y`, but also reverse the signal.
5. Write one line of code to return the first 2 seconds of a monaural wave file imported into matrix `y` with sampling rate `fs`. Assume that the sample is always longer than 2 seconds (i.e., length-checking is not required, as conditionals will be covered in a later section).
6. We have covered one way to switch channels in a stereo sound sample (`fliplr()`). Now, assume that this function does not exist. Write two programs, each demonstrating a different way to switch stereo channels. You may create new variables as necessary.
7. You have an indexing variable `n` and a matrix `M` with `r` rows and `c` columns, where `n` can be any real number from negative to positive infinity (**including** nonintegers). Write one line of code that will index `M`, preventing any indexing errors resulting from exceeding matrix dimensions or failing to use a positive integer.

Flow Control

A critical aspect of programs is the ability to select which action to perform based on a set of conditions. For example, we may want to perform one type of processing on stereo sound files but do something else with monaural files. Furthermore, it may be necessary to continue to perform an operation until a certain condition is met. For example, one might want to select a large number of audio files to process, then exit or return a result when all processing is complete. Techniques for achieving flow control most basically involve the use of conditionals, logical operators, `if` statements, and `switch` statements. Figure 1–9 provides an example of a flowchart, which depicts the control of programming flow as might occur in a typical speech-processing application.

Conditionals and Boolean Logic

Boolean logic, named in honor of George Boole (1815–1864), is based on truth values of 0 and 1. In this system, on which most modern computer operations are based, 0 is interpreted as "false" and 1 as "true." MATLAB relational operators function in accordance with this Boolean logic: they will return 1 if the statement to be evaluated is true, or 0 if it is false:

- `a == b`: `a` is equal to `b`
- `a ~= b`: `a` is **not** equal to `b`
- `a > b`: `a` is greater than `b`
- `a >= b`: `a` is greater than or equal to `b`
- `a < b`: `a` is less than `b`
- `a <= b`: `a` is less than or equal to `b`

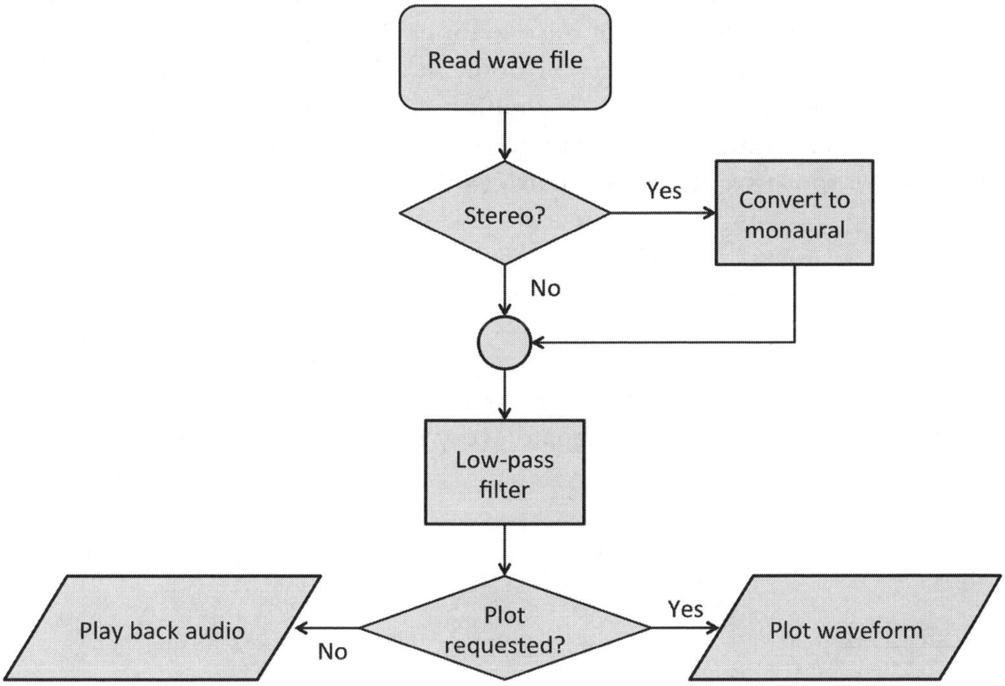

Figure 1–9. Control of programming flowchart.

For example, the tautological statement `5 == 5` will evaluate as true, and therefore return a 1:

```
>> 5 == 5

ans =

1
```

Logical Operators

It is possible to test the truth of multiple statements or propositions simultaneously. For example, we might want to perform a given operation only if a sound sample is longer than 5 seconds AND its RMS amplitude exceeds some value of interest. This can be done with MATLAB's set of logical operators, which take Boolean arguments and return a Boolean truth value:

- `a & b`: both `a` and `b` are true
- `a | b`: either `a` or `b` is true, or both
- `~a`: `a` is **not** true

It is important to understand that these operators can be used on matrices and act in an element-wise manner. The same holds true for logical operators applied to matrices of Boolean values. However, both matrices must be of the same size and orientation. That is to say, for any element-wise operation on matrices `a` and `b`, `size(a)` must be equal to `size(b)`. For example, suppose we have two matrices of Booleans, `a` = `[0 1 0 1]` and `b` = `[0 0 1 1]`:

```
>> a = [0 1 0 1];

>> b = [0 0 1 1];
```

Using the `~` operator will negate every element in the matrix:

```
>> ~a

ans =

   1  0  1  0
```

Using the & operator will return a 1 for every cell whose corresponding cell in **both** matrices is a 1. In this example, only the last element of the result is 1 because only that element corresponds to a 1 in the cells of both of the operands:

```
>> a & b

ans =

  0  0  0  1
```

Finally, using the | operator will return a 1 for any cell where at least one of the corresponding cells in a or b is equal to 1. In this case, all but 1 of the cells are 1, since only 1 cell (the first) contains neither a 1 in matrix a nor a 1 in matrix b:

```
>> a | b

ans =

  0  1  1  1
```

Advanced Use of Conditionals

Because a Boolean value can be represented as a numerical 1 or 0, the result of any of the above conditional operations can be used in a regular mathematical operation, and vice versa. For example, suppose we wanted to define a function that returned x^2 if x>=1, but 1/x if x<1. Without using an if statement, which we will explore next, we could simply write in one line:

```
>> x = 5;

>> y = (x^2) * (x>=1) + (1/x) * (x<1)

y =

  25

>> x = 0.1;

>> y = (x^2) * (x>=1) + (1/x) * (x<1)

y =

  10
```

For example, when the conditional `(x>=1)` is false (i.e., `x` is less than 1), it evaluates to zero, so the entire term `(x^2) * (x>=1)` becomes zeroed out and is not included in the final product: `(x^2) * 0 + (1/x) * (x<1)` becomes `0 + (1/x) * 1` or simply `(1/x)`, as intended.

The `if` Statement

Quite possibly the most used keyword in MATLAB is `if`, which allows the programmer to choose the next course of action depending on other information at hand (i.e., values stored in variables). For example,

```
a = 5;
if a == 5
    disp('The value of a is 5.')
end
```

```
The value of a is 5.
```

In this case, the `disp()` function is only called if the value of `a` is 5. Note that an `if` block must always be terminated with an `end` statement to let MATLAB know where to resume execution after evaluating it. It is possible to construct a series of `if` statements, for example, if there are a number of possible outcomes and separate actions to perform for each one. Here, the series is chained together with the `elseif` keyword, which checks each condition in turn.

```
a = 5;
if a < 5
    disp('The value of a is too small.')
    % e.g. perform corrective operations here.
elseif a == 5
    disp('The value of a is 5. This is correct!')
    % e.g. perform main analysis operations here.
elseif a > 5
    disp('The value of a is too big.')
    % e.g. perform corrective operations here.
end
```

```
The value of a is 5. This is correct!
```

Finally, the `else` statement will tell MATLAB what to do if none of the conditions specified in the `if` or `elseif` statements evaluate to true:

```
a = 10;
if a < 10
    disp('The value of a is less than 10.')
else
    disp('The value of a is greater than or equal to 10.')
end
```

```
The value of a is greater than or equal to 10.
```

For more than three cases, a `switch` statement is preferable. We will now explore the proper usage of this statement.

The `switch` Statement

When testing a large number of possible cases, the `switch` statement offers greater simplicity than a long chain of `if` and `elseif` lines. A `switch` statement starts with the syntax `switch myVar`, where `myVar` may take on any number of values (e.g., not just Boolean). Within the `switch` block, the `case` statement specifies what to do in each case (i.e., each possible value of `myVar`). An `otherwise` statement acts as a catch-all if none of the `case` statements are executed. Finally, as with `if`, the `switch` block ends with the `end` keyword:

```
a = 4;
switch a
    case 3
        disp('The value of a is 3.')
    case 4
        disp('The value of a is 4.')
    case 5
        disp('The value of a is 5.')
    otherwise
        disp('The value of a is neither 3, 4, nor 5. Try again!')
end
```

```
The value of a is 4.
```

If two or more cases are to be executed with the same code, the case values can be included in a cell array:

```
a = 10;
switch a
    case {9, 10, 11}
        disp('The value of a is 9, 10, or 11')
    otherwise
        disp('The value of a is neither 9, 10, nor 11')
end
```

```
The value of a is 9, 10, or 11.
```

Note that it is not convenient (and sometimes impossible) to test relations involving inequality with a `switch` statement; in these cases, an `if` statement is preferred. Observe the difference in the result from a simple grade comparison under the two statements:

```
grade = 95.1;
if grade >= 90
    disp('Congratulations! You earned an A.')
else
    disp('Too bad!')
end
```

```
Congratulations! You earned an A.
```

```
switch grade
    case {90, 91, 92, 93, 94, 95, 96, 97, 98, 99, 100}
        disp('Congratulations! You earned an A.')
    otherwise
        disp('Too bad!')
end
```

```
Too bad!
```

To summarize: if the variable of interest is discrete (i.e., it can take on only a limited set of values), then either `if` or `switch` statements are useful.

If the variable is continuous, then conditionals based on `if` statements are preferable.

Applications

We will now explore several applications of conditionals in speech processing. As before, let us create a sample two-channel audio matrix. This time, we will assume a standard sampling rate `fs = 44100` and generate 2.5 seconds of white-noise audio data:

```
>> fs = 44100;

>> y = rand(fs*2.5, 2)*2-1;
```

The workspace now contains the two variables `y` and `fs`, just as though the command `[y, fs] = audioread('myAudioFile.wav');` had been executed. Suppose we wanted to perform an operation that required 3 seconds of audio. A preliminary check might be written something like this:

```
length_seconds = length(y)/fs
if length_seconds >= 3
    disp('Signal length is acceptable. Performing operation!');
    % (Insert other code here)
else
    disp('Warning! Signal is too short. Cannot continue.')
end
```

```
length_seconds =

    2.5000

Warning! Signal is too short. Cannot continue.
```

Functions

Although MATLAB contains many useful functions such as `sin()`, `sqrt()`, and so on, its real power as a programming language stems from the user's ability to create custom functions and script files, saving a sequence of commonly used commands for later recall. Function-definition syntax and management of `.m` files are detailed, as well as function nesting.

What Is a Function?

In MATLAB, a **function** is a piece of code that will

1. Take some number of arguments, or operands, as input (0 or more).
2. Perform operations on said arguments, including printing messages, generating plots or graphics, or saving files.
3. Return some number of outputs (0 or more).

The simplest possible function is the trivial case of one that takes no arguments, does nothing, and returns nothing. In MATLAB, functions can be defined with the `function` keyword and must be saved in a file with the same name as the function. In the following case, this code would be saved in `do_nothing.m`:

```
function do_nothing()
    % This function does absolutely nothing!
end
```

Calling this function will have no effect on any variables, figures, or files, whatsoever. Let us examine a more useful, but still trivial, bit of code. This next function, `test()`, exhibits the use of both input and output arguments. Input arguments are those that are within the parentheses after the function name—multiple arguments will be separated by commas. Also in the function definition line, notice the equals sign. This is used to let MATLAB know that this function may produce output arguments, which are named to the left of the sign. Assignment to the variable named in the function definition line can be done anywhere in the body of the function, and MATLAB will return the desired result:

```
function y = test(a)
    y = a+1;
end
```

If this function is called with the expression `test(6)`, MATLAB will evaluate it to `7`, storing this value in the default variable `ans` unless another destination variable is explicitly specified:

```
>> test(6)

ans =

     7

>> myVar = test(6);
>> disp(myVar)

  7
```

Multiple input arguments are separated by commas. Suppose we wanted to define a function that returned the product of two numbers, divided by their absolute difference. If we were to call this function `prodOverDiff` and save it in the file `prodOverDiff.m`, the following code would perform the task.

```
function z = prodOverDiff(x, y)
    z = x * y / abs(x - y);
end
```

It is also possible to have multiple output arguments. In this case, the arguments are enclosed in brackets. The following example demonstrates a function that simply swaps the values of two arguments, replicating to some extent the behavior of the built-in `deal()` function.

```
function [x, y] = swap(x, y)
    temp = x;
    x = y;
    y = temp;
end
```

This function would be called as follows:

```
>> x = 1;
>> y = 2;
>> [x, y] = swap(x, y)

x =

     2

y =

     1
```

File Operations

When undertaking any sort of research, one needs to understand processes for data management. Specifically, answers to the following questions will help or improve analysis procedures and programs:

- Where are my data stored relative to my analysis scripts?
- What format(s) are the files in? (This is sometimes, but not always, equivalent to the question, "What are the file extensions?")
- Can I open the files or convert them to a format my program can understand?
- How can I point my analysis programs at the right data files?
- How are the data stored in each file (order of variables)?

In this section, good file management and selection practices are demonstrated, followed by a series of examples focusing on common file types in speech and language research:

- Delimited plain text/ASCII (`.txt` or `.csv`)
- Microsoft Excel (`.xls` or `.xlsx`)
- Audio recording (`.wav` or `.au`)
- Binary data or proprietary formats (for advanced users)

Each module will demonstrate how to open and process data from each of the above formats. Example files can be downloaded from the course website.

File Management and Paths

It is important to review the concept of MATLAB's search path here. There are two types of paths: absolute and relative.

- Absolute paths begin with a drive-letter designation in Windows (e.g., `C:`), or with the root character / in Linux, Unix, and Mac OS X. An example of an absolute path would be something like `C:\Analysis project\data\subject1.txt`.
- Relative paths begin with either a file name or a folder name, and are followed relative to the program or file from which they are referenced.

In MATLAB, when a function is called or a file is opened without an absolute path, MATLAB will first look in the current working directory (i.e., the files shown in the Current Directory window). If a matching file is not found there, MATLAB will then look through the system paths stored in its search path. Call the function path to display MATLAB's current search path, which may vary by platform and version. In this example, the full list is truncated to save space:

```
>> path

          MATLABPATH

     C:\Users\jdvorak\Documents\MATLAB
     C:\Program Files\MATLAB\R2015b\toolbox\matlab\addons
     ...
     ...
     ...
     C:\Program Files\MATLAB\R2015b\toolbox\wavelet\wavelet
     ...
```

You may recall the audioread function, which we have been using quite simply with relative filenames, assuming the file was in the current directory or at least the same folder as the analysis script. Although lumping data files and analysis programs all together in one folder does work, this approach is a bit naive, so we now discuss a more user-friendly and effective approach to opening files.

Using the function uigetfile, we can open a graphical window to allow the user to select files. It is important to note that this function does not return the data from the file(s) itself, but only the path to the file(s)—subsequent functions or commands can then be called with the output of uigetfile as their input arguments, pointing them at the desired file.

Because we do not advocate storing data files in the same folder as the analysis program for any but the simplest cases, it becomes necessary to specify an absolute path for all target files. This is done with the uigetfile function by specifying two output arguments, as follows. Notice that we use the variable name pathName to avoid masking the inbuilt path() function or inadvertently affecting the MATLAB search path:

```
>> [fileName, pathName] = uigetfile();
```

After acquiring these elements, a platform-independent way of recombining them into absolute paths involves the use of the fullfile() function:

```
>> absolutePath = fullfile(pathName, fileName);
```

Our lab uses a function called load_files which is built around uigetfile, but controls for cases where the user aborts, selects the wrong file, selects only one file where multiple files are expected, and so on. This function, along with example code, is available on the companion website at http://www.pluralpublishing.com/publication/mpslpa.

It is now assumed that you are able to supply all subsequent functions with an absolute path to any file desired, either by using `uigetfile`, `load_files`, or a function of your own design.

ASCII Files

In the computing world, plain text using ASCII encoding is often seen as the lowest common denominator. Practically every programming language or major piece of analysis software has some facility for dealing with text files. Specifically, these files are usually of the **delimited** variety, which means that the fields (equivalent to cells in a spreadsheet) are separated within a row by some character (often ,). Naturally, rows are separated by a line break.

In MATLAB scripts, reading text files can be accomplished with the `dlmread` function. Note that `dlmread` works only with text files with *all* numerical data. For reading mixed text/numerical data, we will use another function discussed later. `dlmread` is called with the path to a file as its argument and returns a matrix. By default, this function expects to see the comma used as a delimiter in the file, but will adjust if it detects different delimiters being used (tabs and spaces are common).

One common use of such files is as an interchange format exported from instrumentation software. For example, ASL Eyenal software can export eye data obtained, say, during a sentence-reading task, to a comma-delimited text file.

Excel Files

Excel files are read through the `xlsread()` function. This function returns three arguments, typically called `num`, `txt`, and `raw`. The `num` argument contains all numeric information found, with `NaN` replacing text. The `txt` argument contains the text information, with blanks replacing numeric. Finally, the `raw` argument is a cell array, which can contain different types of elements, and represents the complete spreadsheet.

Another way to read Excel files, and one that will be discussed more in depth in **Chapter 5**, is the `readtable()` function. This converts the data in the file into a `table` object, which is an important precursor to many data-analysis methods.

Audio Files

As discussed earlier, the `audioread()` function can be used to import audio data into MATLAB. A full discussion of this function is postponed until **Chap-**

ter 2, but the essential operations consist of providing a relative or absolute path to a file as an input argument, and acquiring the audio data and sampling rate through output arguments.

A typical call to this function, say to read a file called `'patient1SpeechSample.wav'`, would be along the lines of

```
>> [y, fs] = audioread('patient1SpeechSample.wav');
```

This command will load the audio data into the variable `y`, and the sampling rate (in samples per second) into `fs`.

Proprietary Formats

In many cases, research instruments or software tools save their data in proprietary formats. If the tool of interest does not have a method to export its data into a common interchange format such as Excel, CSV, or plain text, it may be necessary to find or write custom file-importation routines. For some proprietary formats, MATLAB code already exists. As an example, some models of ASL eye trackers save the record of tracked gaze positions in a proprietary `.eyd` format. To read this type of file into MATLAB, one can use the ILAB package (Gitelman, 2002) and convert the data to MATLAB-compatible data types, such as matrices, vectors, and structs.

In the case that packages are unavailable, but the structure of the file is known, one can use low-level file input/output functions to manually acccss the bytes in the file and convert them into MATLAB-usable data. This topic is somewhat beyond the scope of the text, but we will include an example of parsing a simple binary file with a known format.

Suppose we have a sound-pressure level meter and an associated software package that outputs files in a custom format. The first 2 bytes of the file, when interpreted as an integer value, denote the sampling rate. For example, the sequence `03E8` in hexadecimal would correspond to 1,000 samples per second. The remaining bytes of the file indicate the measured SPL at that sample, such that a value of `00` corresponds to a reading of 20 dB, and a value of `FF` corresponds to a reading of 90 dB. We want to create a MATLAB function that reads such a file and then outputs a `y` and `fs` in a manner similar to `audioread()`.

When working with low-level operations, it is necessary to explicitly open and close a file for reading. This is done with the `fopen()` and `fclose()` functions, respectively. Suppose the file of interest is named `mySPLfile.dat`. The code to open this file for binary access is as follows. Note the assignment to a file ID, called `fid`. File IDs are used to keep track of multiple open files and data sources at once:

```
>> fid = fopen('mySPLfile.dat');
```

Once the file is opened in binary mode, it can be read in by using the fread() function. Note that, unlike higher-level file reading functions, fread() requires the file-id fid as an argument, not a file name. In this case, the data are returned as a column vector of values between 0 and 255, inclusive, representing the range of bytes:

```
>> data = fread(fid);
```

After reading in the data, it is good practice to close the file:

```
>> fclose(fid);
```

Now that the data are in a vector, we convert them to meaningful values for clinical examination or data analysis using our knowledge of the file format. The first 2 bytes represent the sampling rate in Hertz, but must be converted to decimal. By virtue of the binary encoding, we can consider the first byte to represent 256 times the place value of the second one. That is, the sequence 0100 would correspond to 256, whereas 0001 would correspond to 1. In MATLAB, we can convert these 2-byte values to a decimal number as follows:

```
>> fs = data(1) * 256 + data(2);
```

We then remove this "header" information from the file and keep only the byte data representing the SPL measurements. To do this, we index into the data vector starting at the third element:

```
>> data = data(3:end);
```

Finally, we are ready to convert the byte values to SPL measurements in decibels. Taking into account the meter range mentioned above (20 to 90 dB), we first compute a decibel-per-unit scaling factor by taking the range in decibels (90 − 20 = 70) and dividing by the range in byte values (255) to get approximately 0.2745:

```
>> scaleFactor = (90 - 20) / 255;
```

After scaling, the values in the vector represent the distance of each sample from the baseline (20 dB). This baseline is then added in as an offset:

```
>> y = data * scaleFactor + 20;
```

Combining the above into a function, saved in `splread.m`, we have

```
function [y, fs] = splread(fileName)

    % Open the file and extract the binary data.
    fid = fopen(fileName);
    data = fread(fid);
    fclose(fid);

    % Use the two-byte header to compute sampling frequency.
    fs = data(1) * 256 + data(2);

    % Remove the header.
    data = data(3:end);

    % Compute scaling factor.
    scaleFactor = (90 - 20) / 255;

    % Convert binary to dB.
    y = data * scaleFactor + 20;

end
```

This can now be used as though it were a built-in function and extends the range of MATLAB's capability to our hypothesized instrument:

```
>> [y, fs] = splread('mySPLfile.dat');
>> y(1:5)

ans =

 36.4706
 36.7451
 37.8431
 35.6471
 37.2941

>> fs

fs =

    1000
```

References

Gitelman, D. R. (2002). ILAB: A program for postexperimental eye movement analysis. *Behavior Research Methods, Instruments, and Computers, 34*(4), 605–612.

Guenther, F. H., Ghosh, S. S., & Tourville, J. A. (2006). Neural modeling and imaging of the cortical interactions underlying syllable production. *Brain and Language, 96*, 280–301.

Klatt, D. H. (1980). Software for a cascade/parallel formant synthesizer. *Journal of the Acoustical Society of America, 67*(3), 971–995.

2

Basic Operations for Sampling and Wave Data

Sampling: Analog Signals to Digital Data

In speech, language, and hearing research and clinical practice, one of the most commonly used file types is `.wav`, which serves as a container for audio data. Examples of data stored in this format could be patient speech samples, results from articulation tests, or even data collected during experimental tasks. Here we draw an important distinction between ideal mathematics and practical application. We consider the functional form of the longitudinal sound-pressure wave that composes human speech to be real valued; that is, between any two pressure values it is possible to find a third, no matter how close the two are to each other. Similarly, between any two points in time we can find a third. However, as discussed earlier, computers and storage devices have finite precision, memory, and storage capacities. In order to capture a continuous audio signal from the external world and digitize it in a manner that allows storage and later retrieval on a digital, binary device, the wave must be *sampled.*

Sampling consists of taking a measurement of a quantity, in this case air pressure, at a specified rate and to a specified precision. Readers may be familiar with the number 44100 Hz, which is the *sampling rate* for CD-quality audio. This means that the continuous-time signal from the human voice or other audio source is measured 44100 times per second. The sampling precision for audio is usually 16-bit, meaning that a range of 65536 (equaling 2^{16}) values can be used to represent pressure measurements. For completeness, we mention that several different encoding and representation schemes are available to make the most of this range of numbers, but fortunately MATLAB automatically detects and uses the correct scheme when reading and writing a `.wav` file.

Thus, the quality of a sampled signal relies on two sampling parameters: rate and precision. Increasing the sampling rate allows finer-grained time distinctions to be made but has no effect on distinguishing one value of the signal from a similar value. On the other hand, increasing sampling precision allows for finer separation of close measurements of the signal, but has no effect on improving temporal resolution. In both cases, higher precision leads to greater file sizes. For example, 1 minute of speech sampled at 44.1 kHz and digitized with 16-bit precision will take up 44100 samples/sec × 60 sec × 16 bits/sample × 1 byte/8 bits = 5,292,000 bits, or approximately 5 megabytes. For this reason, a variety of compression schemes and corresponding file formats, such as `.mp3`, `.flac`, `.mp4`, and `.ogg`, have been devised. All of these formats are readable in MATLAB through use of the `audioread()` function.

In Figure 2–1 are reproduced two different samplings of a "speech signal" (actually a simple 3-Hz sine wave for purposes of clarity) with sampling rate indicated. Notice how the higher sampling rate allows better reconstruction of the original signal.

Note that, strictly speaking, the discrete points of this sampled signal should not be connected, but we do so to highlight the contrast in quality.

In the above two examples, we have allowed the sampling *precision* to be as large as possible within the limits of MATLAB's floating-point representation, which is in fact quite a bit higher than that found in a standard `.wav` file. In Figure 2–2 are reproduced two different samplings of the same signal, but with drastically different precisions. These were simulated by multiplying the signal by a given power of 2 to represent the number of bits, then rounding the result and dividing back.

The reader may be tempted to ask, "Is there some sampling rate below which the signal cannot be reproduced?" To answer this we turn to the Nyquist-Shannon sampling theorem (Nyquist, 1928; Shannon, 1949), which states that one must sample at least twice as fast as the frequency of interest in order to represent this frequency in the signal. Alternatively, this theorem states that the maximum frequency detectable under a given sampling rate, say `fs`, is equal to `0.5*fs`, known as the Nyquist frequency or folding frequency, denoted `fn`. In MATLAB, one can easily compute this frequency:

```
>> fn = 0.5 * fs;
```

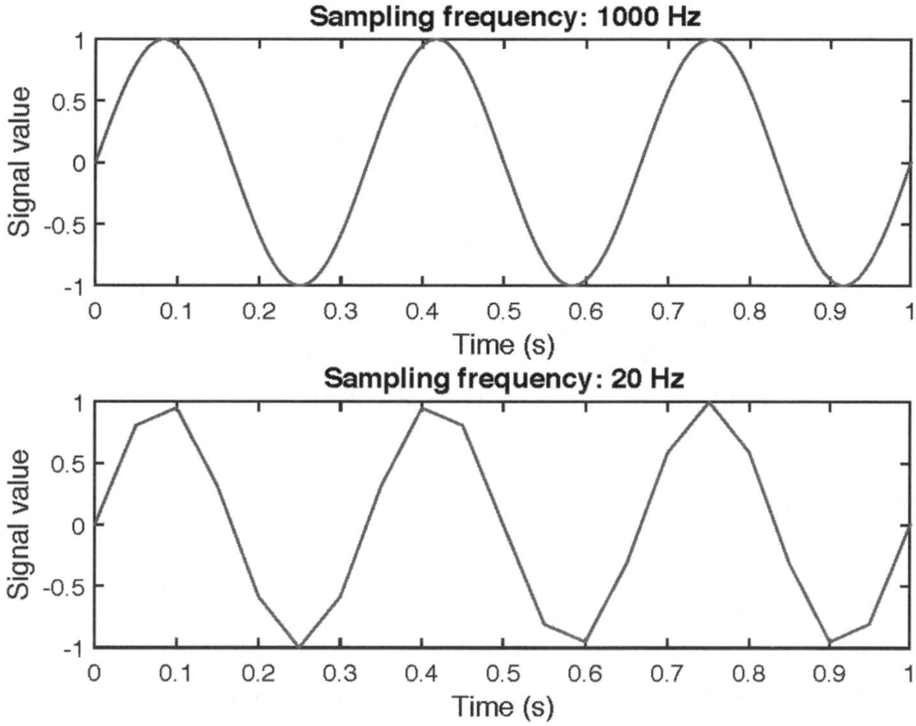

Figure 2–1. Speech signal sampled at different sampling rates.

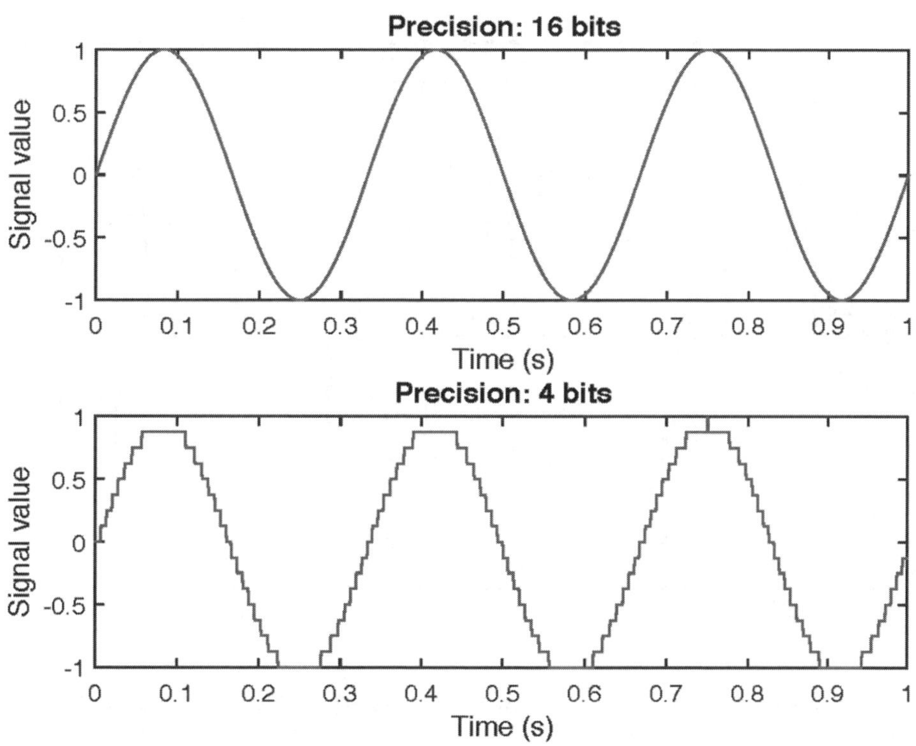

Figure 2–2. Speech signal sampled with different sampling precisions.

Figure 2–3 demonstrates the effect of sampling at too low a rate to capture a certain frequency. We simulate an original analog signal (continuous waveform) including a combination of a 3-Hz and 20-Hz tone, which is sampled (vertical lines) by an instrument capable of 30 samples per second. By the Nyquist–Shannon theorem, the 20-Hz tone will not be adequately captured by this instrument, whose maximum detectable frequency is 15 Hz. Unfortunately, this higher-frequency component does not simply disappear but is in fact represented incorrectly as a frequency under the Nyquist limit (one half the sampling frequency). This phenomenon is known as *aliasing* and can prove detrimental to signal quality if not properly addressed. It is for this reason high-speed measurement instruments often include antialiasing filters, which remove frequencies higher than the Nyquist limit before sampling.

Fortunately for speech researchers, these filters are also built into most common recording devices and sound cards. Furthermore, unless the sampling rate is set quite low (e.g., under 8 kHz), we need not be too concerned about the Nyquist limit when investigating frequency ranges of interest for speech (approximately 50–300 Hz for voice pitch, and approximately 500–5000 Hz for formants).

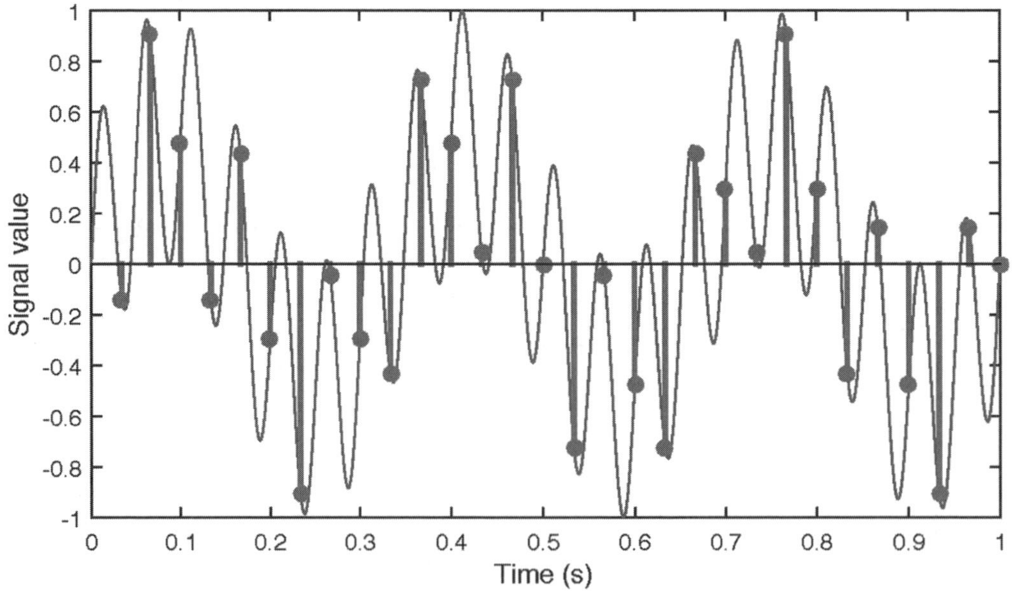

Figure 2–3. Analog signal sampled with insufficient sampling frequency under the Nyquist–Shannon theorem.

Reading Sampled Data into MATLAB®

A strength of MATLAB is its facility in loading `.wav` files and numerous other common formats without requiring the user to master low-level operating system file commands. Importing wave data from a therapy session or experimental response can be accomplished with one line of code:

```
>> y = audioread('myWave.wav');
```

Be sure to include the semicolon (`;`) in this command to suppress the result of evaluating the `audioread()` function. Otherwise, the Command Window will be filled with the numerical representation of the wave data imported, possibly containing thousands of rows.

Note that this command returns only the samples themselves, with no information on rate or precision. This is fine if there is agreement beforehand on the sampling rate to use. However, if the rate is unknown, the following command structure is preferred:

```
>> [y, fs] = audioread('myWave.wav');
```

This code uses multiple output arguments, which we explored in the subsection on functions. Here, the actual data are assigned to `y`, and the sampling rate (samples per second) is assigned to `fs`. The `audioread()` function has been designed so that both of the following are legal calls:

```
>> y = audioread('myWave.wav');
>> [y, fs] = audioread('myWave.wav');
```

That is to say, `fs` is an *optional* output argument. Similarly to optional input arguments, optional output arguments must be specified in order, and later arguments cannot be requested without also including earlier ones.

If it is known in advance how many samples are to be read, an optional input argument can be used. The start and stop points are specified in a two-element row vector, in samples. For example, suppose we only want to read the first second of a file and know in advance that the sampling rate is 44100 Hz and that the file exceeds 1 second in length. This can be accomplished as follows:

```
>> yFirst = audioread('myWave.wav', [1, 44100]);
```

If we do not know the sampling rate in advance, we can query the file without fully loading the audio data by means of the `audioinfo()` function. This function returns a structure with fields corresponding to pertinent audio properties. Structure fields are accessed with dot notation, which is demonstrated in the example below. This example assumes we want the first 500 ms of the file, and that the file exceeds 500 ms in length:

```
>> info = audioinfo('myWave.wav');
>> finalSample = round(500 * info.SampleRate / 1000);
>> yFirst = audioread('myWave.wav', [1, finalSample]);
```

Working With Audio Files

Understanding Wave Data

When MATLAB opens a `.wav` file, the binary values are interpreted as signed floating-point numbers (doubles) ranging from –1 to 1. This is the normalized voltage generated by the sound card used to record the data, and unfortunately has little bearing on the actual sound amplitude or sound pressure level. A common beginner's question is "How do I determine the sound pressure level in dB from this file?" Unfortunately, without detailed information on the calibration of the microphone and sound card settings used, this is generally impossible. The recorded voltage can depend on microphone settings, the sound card used, and even the volume level chosen beforehand.

However, other useful information can still be obtained without calibration. In Chapter 4, we will cover simple methods of fundamental-frequency extraction, amplitude envelope generation for prosodic calculations, and spectral analyses for formant detection, among other techniques.

In MATLAB, the matrix generated by `audioread()` will have numerous rows and either one or two columns, representing monaural or stereo data, respectively. If a file is stereo, column 1 represents the left channel and column 2 the right.

Many MATLAB functions that are designed for signal processing will also expect their inputs to be in this format; that is to say, they operate *column-wise*. When accessing an element of this audio matrix, recall that each row represents a sample, not a second or millisecond. The actual amount of time each sample takes up is dependent on the sampling rate used; this is why sampling-rate information is included in most audio file formats.

Examining Waveforms

With a matrix y and sampling rate fs imported successfully into MATLAB, one might wish to examine the waveform. Here we make use of the plot() function, but special care must be taken to create an appropriate vector of times in seconds, milliseconds, or whatever unit is desired. Using the range operator (:), one can write an expression to generate an appropriate time vector as follows:

```
>> time = (1:length(y)) / fs;
```

A useful side effect of this approach is that the last element of time will also correspond to the length of the audio data in seconds. To plot the signal by its appropriate time vector, use

```
>> plot(time, y)
>> xlabel('Time (s)')
>> ylabel('Y')
```

This will result in something resembling Figure 2–4.

Playing Sounds From Wave Data

There are a variety of ways to play wave data in MATLAB. One can make use of the sound() or soundsc() functions, or create an audioplayer object. The latter option is recommended in the latest version of MATLAB. In all cases, the sampling rate should be supplied or MATLAB will default to a given sampling frequency, usually 8 kHz. We will now discuss the merits and drawbacks of each approach.

The sound() function is relatively simple but does not scale the output at all, even if it is beyond the range of ±1. This may result in unpleasant clipping if the data have not been range-checked before playback. A waveform stored in y, with sampling rate fs, can be played by entering the following command:

```
>> sound(y, fs)
```

The soundsc() function, on the other hand, will scale all data points, even those which are already within the ±1 range. Although this prevents

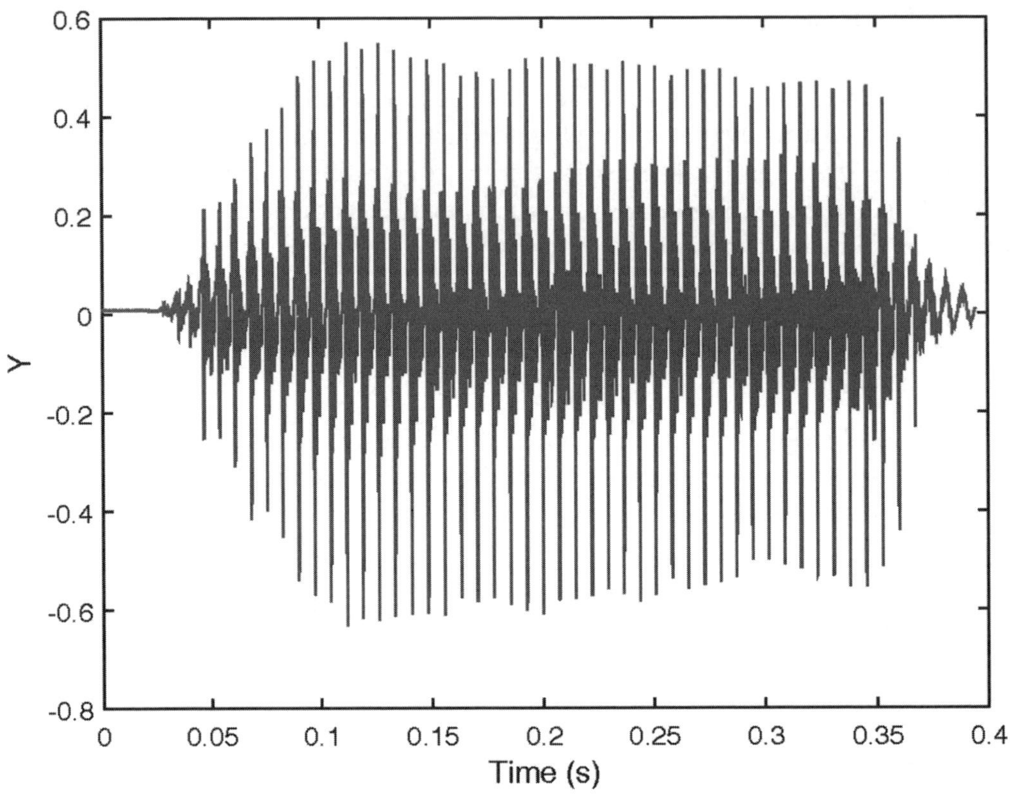

Figure 2–4. Waveform plot.

the type of clipping that can occur with `sound()`, it may result in unintended amplification of a low-volume file. Usage is identical to the `sound()` function:

```
>> soundsc(y, fs)
```

Finally, an `audioplayer` object encapsulates the sound data and metadata in a single object. Unlike simpler variables and structs, objects in MATLAB have their own methods, or functions, associated with them. Although a full exploration of object-oriented programming is beyond the scope of this text, the approach is convenient for audio files in that it helps organize data. A sound loading and playing program might look something like this:

```
>> [y, fs] = audioread('myWave.wav');
>> ap = audioplayer(y, fs);
>> play(ap);
```

In short,

- `sound()`: Use for data that you know are within ±1. This should apply to most .wav files.
- `soundsc()`: Use for data that may lie outside ±1 (e.g., from transformations or other processing) to avoid clipping.
- `audioplayer`: Use to encapsulate the waveform and metadata into a single object.

Saving Wave Files

Having performed one's desired operations on a piece of audio data, it is often desirable to save the result back to a file on disk for later access. This is especially the case when preparing auditory stimuli for an experiment so that the results can be loaded quickly and without the need for recalculation. Saving a matrix of audio data to a file is done with the `audiowrite()` function as follows:

```
>> audiowrite(filename, y, fs)
```

Here, `y` is the audio matrix or column vector stored in a MATLAB variable, `fs` is the desired sampling rate, and `filename` is the desired file name, which may contain a relative or absolute path. In the case where bit precision needs to be specified, one can use the name-value pair argument `BitsPerSample`, as follows, where `nBits` reflects the bit precision desired:

```
>> audiowrite(filename, y, fs, 'BitsPerSample', nBits)
```

Note the lack of semicolon for this function call—this is because `audiowrite()` does not return a value, but instead has the side effect of creating a file in the location specified.

Exercises

1. How do digital signals stored on a computer differ from analog signals in the "real world"? Is it possible to perfectly store a real-world signal on a computer? Why or why not?
2. What might a digital signal with only 1 bit of precision look like?
3. Suppose you are sampling audio data at 1000 Hz. Assume appropriate antialiasing filters are in place. What can be said about the resulting

signal in regard to comprehensibility, given that human speech sounds tend to range from 75 to 10000 Hz? Why?

4. Write a short program to plot only the right channel of a given signal y. Assume that this signal has been previously loaded with the command `[y, fs] = audioread('mySignal.wav');`, but the wave file in question may be a monaural file. Be sure that this plot includes a proper time scale on the *x*-axis. For this exercise, the *y*-axis need not be labeled.
5. You have been tasked with creating an audio-player program that will plot and play a selected clip from a larger file. Allow the user to select a file using a graphical user interface, preferably with `uigetfile()`. Using any input method we have discussed so far (e.g., command-line input or dialog boxes), ask the user for the starting and stopping time in milliseconds. Check that these times are valid numbers and within the range of the data, and report an error to the user if anything goes wrong. Create a complete plot with appropriate axis labels, a descriptive title incorporating the name of the file, and time units in milliseconds. Finally, play back the selected region of the file, checking for appropriate amplitude range to avoid clipping.
6. Complete **Exercise 5**, but instead of plotting and playing the wave data, save the waveform to disk as a new file. Use `uiputfile()` to allow the user to specify the desired output file name. Be sure to save the file with the same sampling frequency and bit precision as the original.
7. Simulate a "real-world" analog signal by synthesizing a set of sine waves at a high sampling frequency (say 100000 Hz). These waves should have frequencies of 100, 200, 500, and 750 Hz. Sum these waves to create a complex tone. Sample this tone at both 44100 Hz (standard CD-audio rate) and 1000 Hz and comment on the signal and playback quality for both rates.
8. Explore the effects of differing sampling rates on the representation (aliasing) of a high-frequency signal. Write a function that accepts a tone frequency and sampling rate and then plots the reconstructed signal sampled at the specified rate.

Working With Audio Vectors and Matrices

As mentioned in **Chapter 1**, when a `.wav` file is imported into MATLAB, it is represented as either a column vector or a matrix. Column vectors are used to represent monaural data, whereas matrices are used to represent stereo or multichannel data. In an audio matrix, each column represents a separate channel, with column 1 typically denoting the left channel and column 2 the right channel.

Indexing

It is not always necessary to use the entirety of a recording for speech analysis. Often, the signal of interest is sandwiched between periods of silence that can be safely removed. When working with a column vector, this can be done using simple ranged indexing expressions. For example, suppose we have the column vector `y` representing a monaural sound, where `fs` equals 44100 Hz, and we wish to extract the period of time from 1500 to 8500 ms (a sample lasting for 7 seconds). We wish to save the cropped signal to the variable `ySpeech`. To do this, we first convert the start and end times from milliseconds to samples, and then round them off to determine the appropriate indexes to use:

```
>> startSample = round(1500 * fs / 1000);
>> stopSample = round(8500 * fs / 1000);
>> ySpeech = y(startSample:stopSample);
```

For stereo files, the situation is somewhat more complex. In addition to specifying the sample numbers, we must specify the channels of interest. This requires indexing both the row and column number in matrix notation, as described in **Chapter 1**. Just as we can use the colon notation to build a range of sample numbers, so too can we use it to select a range of channels. Suppose we wish to repeat the above cropping operation but are now working with a stereo audio file. Therefore, `y` is now a matrix with two columns. Notice that the row indices come before column indices in the indexing expression, consistent with mathematical notation:

```
>> startSample = round(1500 * fs / 1000);
>> stopSample = round(8500 * fs / 1000);
>> ySpeech = y(startSample:stopSample, 1:2);
```

In the case where the number of columns may not be known beforehand, a shorthand method exists to select all columns in the matrix. This is achieved by using the colon operator on its own, as in the following assignment. In our example, this line can be substituted for the previous final line with identical results:

```
>> ySpeech = y(startSample:stopSample, :);
```

Channel Operations

Depending on one's recording and presentation setup, it may be necessary to convert a mono audio signal to stereo, or vice versa. The first operation is facilitated by the `repmat()` function, which allows one to replicate a matrix (hence the name) a given number of times in the vertical and horizontal dimensions. Supposing we have a column vector `y` containing a mono audio signal, we can easily convert this to a stereo signal (with the same audio in both channels) as follows. Note that, just as with matrix indexing, `repmat()` requires the user to specify the vertical dimension (rows) first, then the horizontal dimension (columns). Here we only want one vertical copy of the matrix (we do not want to repeat the sound), but two horizontal copies (we do want two channels):

```
>> yStereo = repmat(y, 1, 2);
```

In contrast to the above simple operation, conversion from stereo to monaural is somewhat more involved because of the variety of scenarios possible. Depending on the clinical or laboratory setup, one may wish to (a) select a single channel or (b) compute and use the mean of both channels. The first scenario can be done with matrix indexing as follows, again assuming our audio data are stored in the matrix `y`. Here we use the empty colon operator as a shorthand to tell MATLAB to select all rows, and separate the stereo audio matrix into two column vectors for the left and right channel, respectively:

```
>> yLeft = y(:, 1);
>> yRight = y(:, 2);
```

The second scenario can be carried out in two ways. If we know in advance that there are two channels, we can simply compute the mean manually:

```
>> yMean = (y(:, 1) + y(:, 2)) / 2;
```

A more elegant method, and one that is likely more computationally efficient, is to use the built-in `mean()` function and supply a dimension argument. On its own, `mean()` computes the column-wise mean, which is only of interest to determine DC offsets (i.e., whether the signal is systematically higher than the zero point). To compute the row-wise mean, a dimension argument of 2 is supplied. Note that this 2 indicates that means are to be computed along the second dimension of the matrix (columns), and it has nothing to do with the fact that there are two channels. The following statement works for a matrix with any number of channels, even one, and can be used as a preprocessing step when this number is unknown in advance:

```
>>yMean = mean(y, 2);
```

The above operations, of course, assume that one is working with column vectors. However, some waveform synthesis functions and code may output row vectors instead. For example, suppose we used the `linspace` function to construct a sequence of 10,000 increasing radian values from zero to 2π, and then computed a 200-Hz sine wave therefrom:

```
>> theta = linspace(0, 2*pi, 10000);
>> y = sin(200*theta);
```

In this case, `y` would be a 1-by-10,000 matrix (i.e., a row vector). To convert this to a column vector, we would need to transpose it using one of the following two methods:

```
>> yTransposed = transpose(y); % Method 1
>> yTransposed = y'; % Method 2
```

One other method that can be used to solve this problem (without conditional processing), supposing that we know our code will receive a monaural vector, but do not know in advance whether it will be a row or column vector, is to use the colon operator in indexing as follows:

```
>> yColumn = y(:); % Reshape to column vector
```

Amplification

Amplification and attenuation can be accomplished quite easily in MATLAB through scalar multiplication. However, one must be cautious to avoid clipping if the scalar multiplier causes values in the signal to exceed ±1. Suppose we have a signal `y`, which we wish to amplify by a factor of `c`. The code to perform this is quite simple and does not depend on the dimensions of `y` (mono vs. stereo). Note the placement of `c` before `y` in the following expression, consistent with the conventions of matrix multiplication (see Appendix C):

```
>> yAmp = c*y;
```

If `c` is greater than 1, the signal is amplified. If `c` is less than 1, the signal is attenuated. Trivially, if `c` is zero, then the signal is silenced.

Suppose we wish to scale a signal such that its maximum absolute amplitude (i.e., deviation from zero) is equal to 1. This represents the maximum amplification of the raw, unfiltered signal that can be achieved without clipping. The scaling coefficient `c` can be computed by determining the present maximum absolute amplitude and then simply multiplying by its reciprocal. This is effectively equivalent to the following command:

```
>> yMaxed = y / max(abs(y));
```

This approach works for waveforms with amplitudes exceeding 1, as well as for waveforms of lower amplitudes. In fact, the `soundsc()` function discussed earlier performs an essentially identical operation before playback but leaves the original data untouched.

Exercises

1. Write a function that, given a file name, will play the last 500 ms of the file. Use conditional processing/flow control to check whether the file exceeds 500 ms in length. If it does not, the function should play the entire file.
2. Suppose that data have been collected during an articulation screening. For each patient, we know there are approximately 2 seconds of silence between the beginning of the recording and the onset of speech. We wish to automate the removal of this silent period as a preprocessing step for later analysis. Write a function that allows the selection of multiple files using `uigetfile()`, removes the first 2000 milliseconds (remember to check each file's sampling rate), and saves the result into a new file with the string "-trimmed" added to the end of the filename, but before the extension. For example, the file "patient123.wav" would be trimmed and saved as "patient123-trimmed.wav." Use the `fileparts()` function to access the file name components, and the `fullfile()` function to recombine them in a platform-independent manner.

Simple Signal Operations

The above sections have mainly concerned how to get an audio signal into a desired format or location. We now assume that the signal of interest is monaural and stored in a column vector, and address a variety of simple signal-processing techniques that could be used in the preprocessing step of a speech analysis algorithm.

Smoothing

In capturing audio, it is possible that incidental noise may produce clicks or pops in the data. These are represented as spikes in the waveform (Figure 2–5) and can yield erroneous results if not removed or adjusted.

A common approach to removing these jumps is smoothing, in which the overall signal is preserved, but high-frequency transients such as the one in Figure 2–5 are removed. One simple method of smoothing is to perform moving-window averaging on the data. Using this method, a window of a predetermined radius is slid across the signal, with the average of all elements within the window being stored at the corresponding window-center location in a new signal. An example of an equally weighted, three-element moving average is depicted in Figure 2–6.

Even though it is possible to perform the above using loops and iteration (and in fact provides a good programming exercise), it is more practical to apply a process known as convolution (discussed in greater detail in

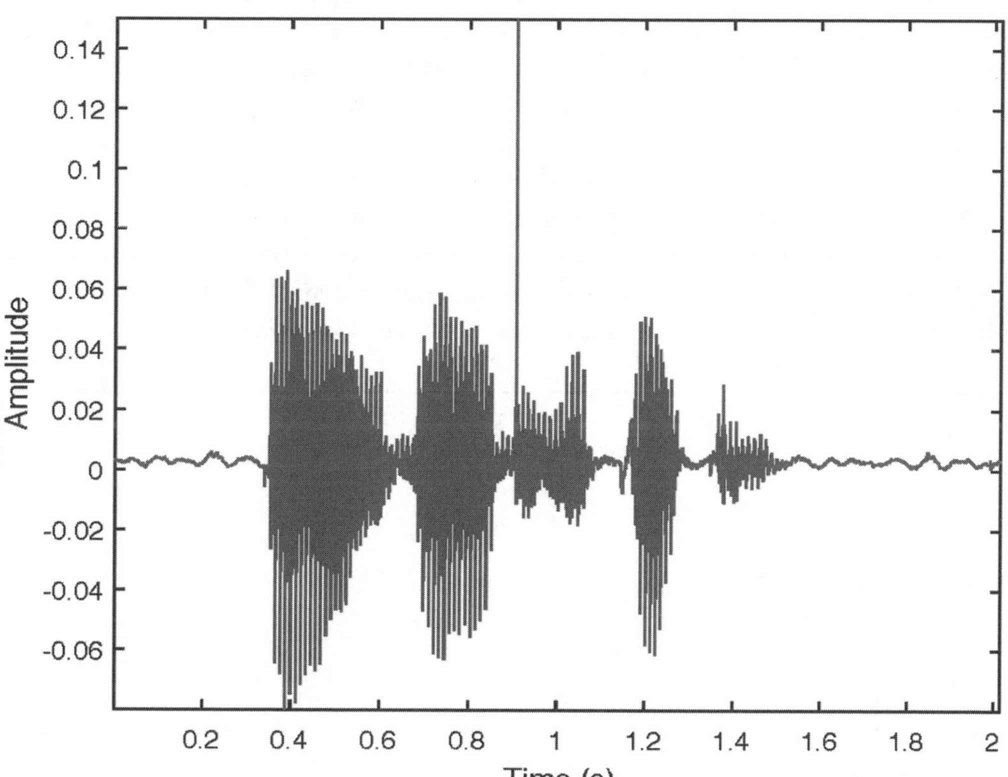

Figure 2–5. Waveform plot with incidental background noise.

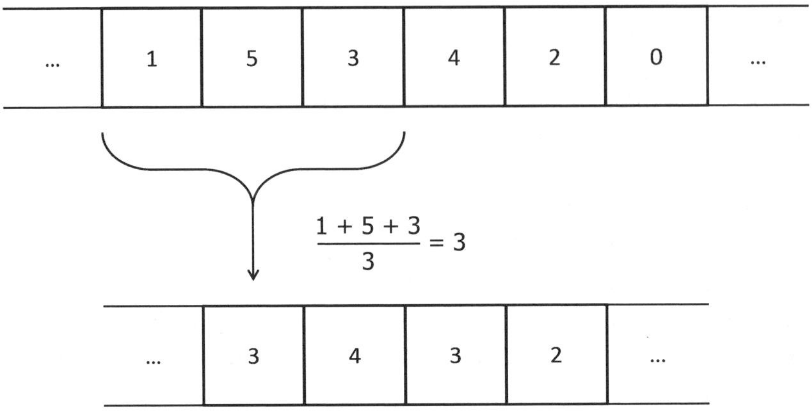

Figure 2–6. Equally weighted, three-element moving average.

Chapter 4). To use convolution for moving-window averaging, one needs to supply the original signal, say `y`, and the window specification, say `w`, to the MATLAB function `conv`. In addition, to ensure that the smoothed signal is the same length as the original one, one must pass in the optional parameter `'same'`. The window specification is simply the factor by which each element of the average is multiplied. For an equally weighted moving average as depicted above, the window is simply n repetitions of the quantity $1/n$, where n is the window length (defined as $2r + 1$, where r is the window radius). The example below applies an 11-element moving-window average (radius = 5) to the data (Figure 2–7). Note the use of the `repmat` function to replicate the scaling factor, and the programmatic specification of the window radius and subsequent computation of window size:

Listing 2–1

```
% Define window radius and size.
r = 5;
winLength = 2*r+1;

% Construct window.
w = repmat(1/winLength, winLength, 1);

% Apply convolution.
ySmoothed = conv(y, w, 'same');
```

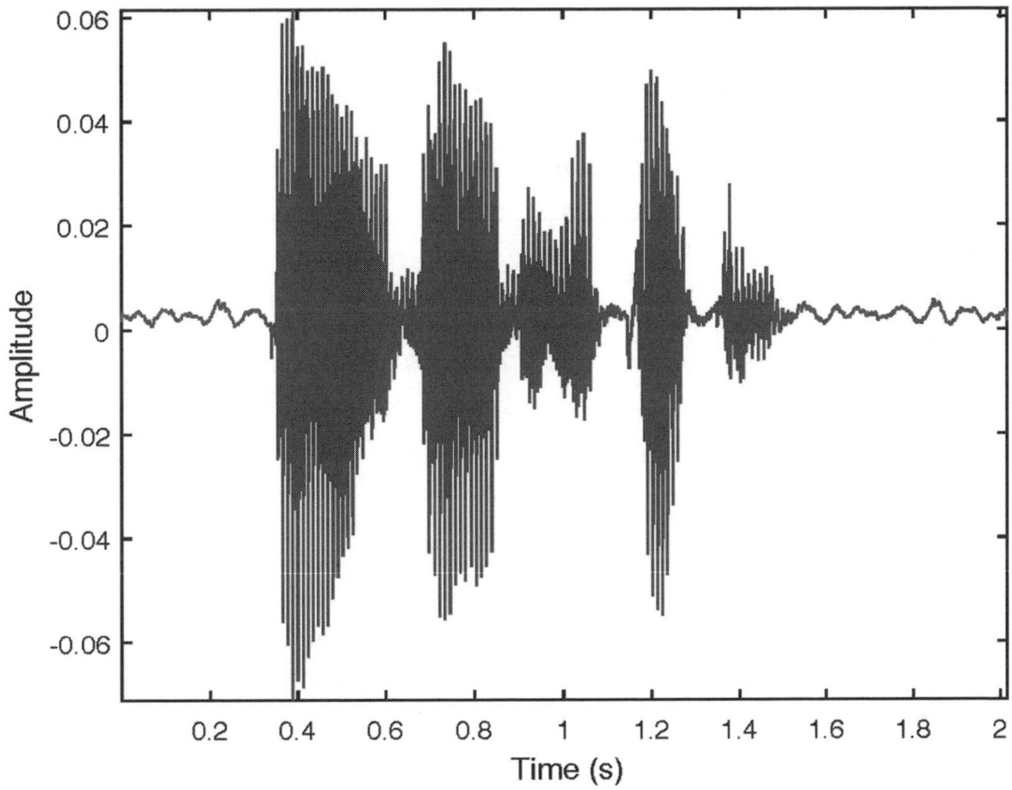

Figure 2–7. Waveform: moving average applied.

```
% Plot results.
time_s = (1:length(ySmoothed))/fs;
plot(time_s, ySmoothed)
axis tight
xlabel('Time (s)')
ylabel('Amplitude')
```

Windowing

Windowing is the process of multiplying each sample in a signal by the value of some windowing function, which is defined over the sample numbers and typically takes values between zero and 1. A common application of windowing is to "taper off" a sound and avoid clicks at the onset and offset, as might occur when presenting, say, a sine tone or white noise. As such, many windowing functions take on a bell-like shape. A variety of windowing functions, defined on the sample numbers 1–100, are depicted in Figure 2–8, with the generating code above. These functions are included in the Signal Processing Toolbox; however, it is possible for users to specify their own windows through custom functions defined in `.m` files (see **Chapter 1**):

Listing 2–2

```
% Define number of points.
n = 100;

% Create a variety of windows for comparison.
w1 = rectwin(n);
w2 = triang(n);
w3 = gausswin(n);
w4 = hamming(n);
```

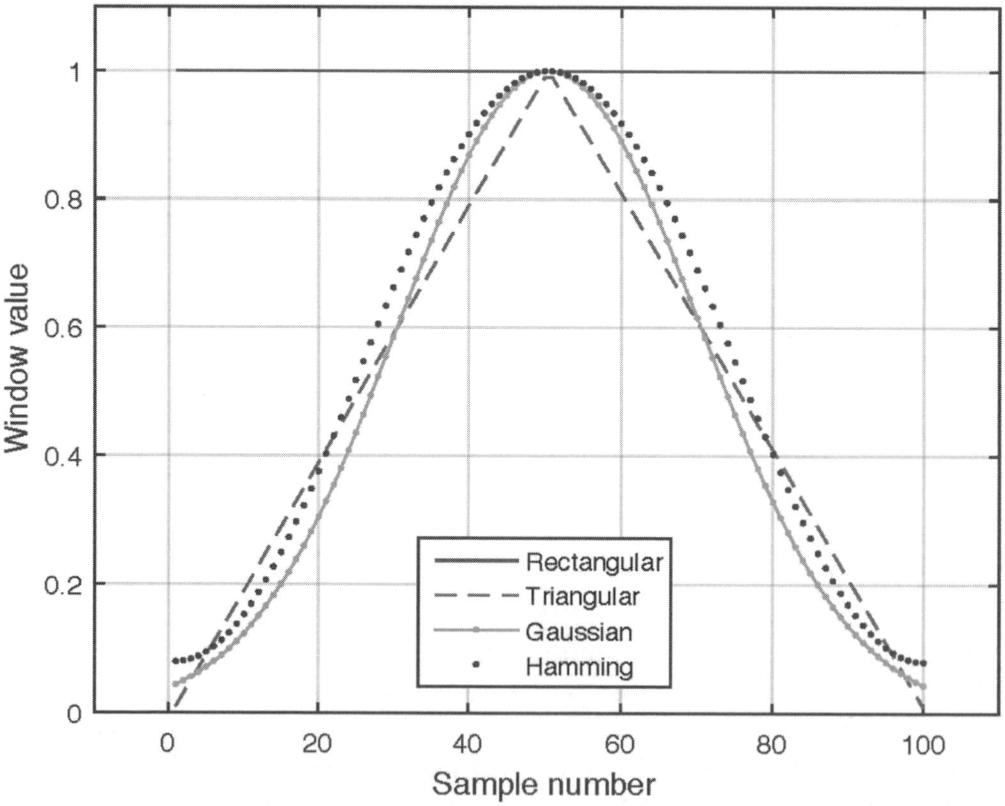

Figure 2–8. Windowing functions,

```
% Plot each window.
plot(w1)
hold on
plot(w2, '--')
plot(w3, '.-')
plot(w4, '.')
hold off

% Add axis labels.
xlabel('Sample number')
ylabel('Window value')

% Add grid.
grid on

% Set up limits so extents of windows are not obscured by axes.
xlim([-10, n+10])
ylim([0, 1.1])

% Add legend at bottom-center position.
legend({'Rectangular', 'Triangular', 'Gaussian', 'Hamming'}, ...
  'Location', 'South');
```

The application of windows to a signal has effects beyond simply changing the amplitude; depending on the window design, the spectrum of the signal may be altered as well. To visualize the effect of a given window, one can use the Window Visualization Tool by means of the `wvtool` function. Although a complete discussion of window design and the visualization tool is beyond the scope of this text, an example is provided in Figure 2–9, comparing a rectangular window (thin line) and a Hamming window (thick line).

Acquisition and Analysis of Nonacoustic Signals Along With Acoustic Signals

The aforementioned techniques pertaining to the acquisition and analysis of sound-wave signals also apply to the acquisition of nonacoustic signals. Whereas in acoustic signals the microphone transduces the signals from pressure to electricity, other transducers commonly used in speech and hearing

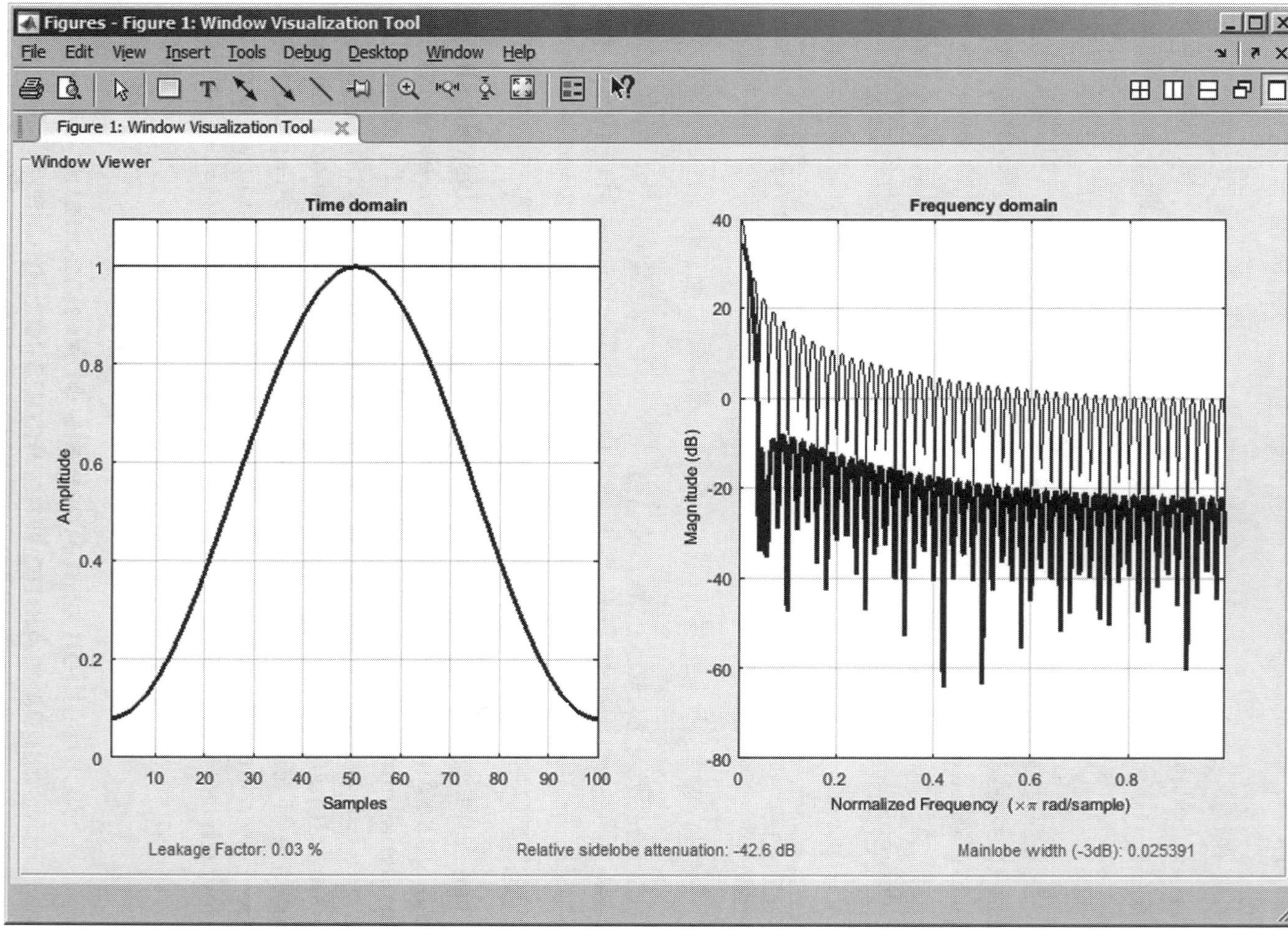

Figure 2–9. Example session of the Window Visualization Tool.

applications likewise change their respective input modality into electrical signals that can be digitized alongside the speech signal or in their own fashion. For example, magnets employed in the Carstens Electromagnetic Articulograph (EMA) and NDI Wave System transduce motion into an electrical signal, while pressure and flow transducers (e.g., Rothenberg mask), strain gauges, and load cells convert air pressure, airflow, and mechanical force into electricity. These transducers are often used to record and quantify articulator kinematics as well as aerodynamical processes along with the speech signal. In addition to these transducers, electrodes can be employed to convert brain (EEG) and/or muscle activity (face, larynx) into electrical activity. The electroglottograph is perhaps most widely used in speech pathology clinics and research applications, and uses electrodes placed on the neck to capture impedance change across the glottis as it opens and closes during phonation. The glottal wave thus obtained easily allows quantification of voice quality through indices including open and closed quotients. Finally, cameras (e.g., video recorders, eye trackers, stroboscopes) transduce light into electrical activity (i.e., a video signal) and can be used to record and quantify movement in the face and larynx. One particular application of cameras in behavioral research is the recording of a participant's eye movements in response to experimental stimuli, also known as eye tracking.

Although it is beyond the scope of this text to explore each of the above devices in detail, some general comments and techniques are useful when analyzing such data alongside audio signals. We have previously mentioned the common audio sampling rate of 44,100 Hz. Unfortunately, it is common for transducers and other equipment to use a variety of sampling rates, ranging from 60 Hz (common for video) to 1 MHz (e.g., for slow-motion Articulograph recordings). This variety necessitates resampling or conversion if, say, a kinematic waveform is to be displayed and analyzed alongside its acoustic counterpart. The following listing demonstrates a typical resampling process in MATLAB, which uses the `resample()` function from the Signal Processing Toolbox, and plots the acoustic and kinematic data side-by-side. For this example, we assume that the acoustic signal in the variable `y` is sampled at 44,100 Hz (`fs`), and the kinematic data `yk` are sampled at `fsk` samples per second. These variables may have been generated from loading external files, or from querying an attached device using the Data Acquisition Toolbox, among other methods. We wish to upsample the kinematic data to match the recorded speech sample.

Listing 2–3. Resampling and Plotting Kinematic Data in MATLAB

```
yk2 = resample(yk, fs, fsk);
time = (1:length(y)) / fs;
timek = (1:length(yk2)) / fs;
figure;
subplot(2,1,1)
plot(time, y)
ylabel('Audio signal')
subplot(2,1,2)
plot(timek, yk2)
ylabel('Kinematic signal')
xlabel('Time (s)');
```

An important assumption of the `resample()` function is that the vector being resampled returns to zero before and after the data. This is a reasonable assumption for audio data because the signal ultimately represents deviations from baseline atmospheric pressure (indicated as 0), but it may not hold for airflow, force, or positional measurements, to name a few. In such cases, it may be more advisable to resample through interpolation using the `spline()` or `interp1()` functions. This is because `resample()` can introduce edge effects when the signal deviates from zero at its endpoints (in Figure 2–10, deviations are indicated with asterisks), as kinematic or positional data often do. For example, positional data in multiple dimensions may use a coordinate system in which the articulators are located in the positive quadrant or octant, preventing return to the true zero point.

Furthermore, spline interpolation generally results in a smooth curve, which is amenable to further operations such as differentiation (e.g., as might be done to estimate instantaneous articulator movement speed).

Listing 2–4. Cubic Spline Interpolation of a Signal

```
% Simulate signal without zero as baseline.
t = 0:10;
y = cos(t) + 2;

% Plot original signal.
stem(t, y)
```

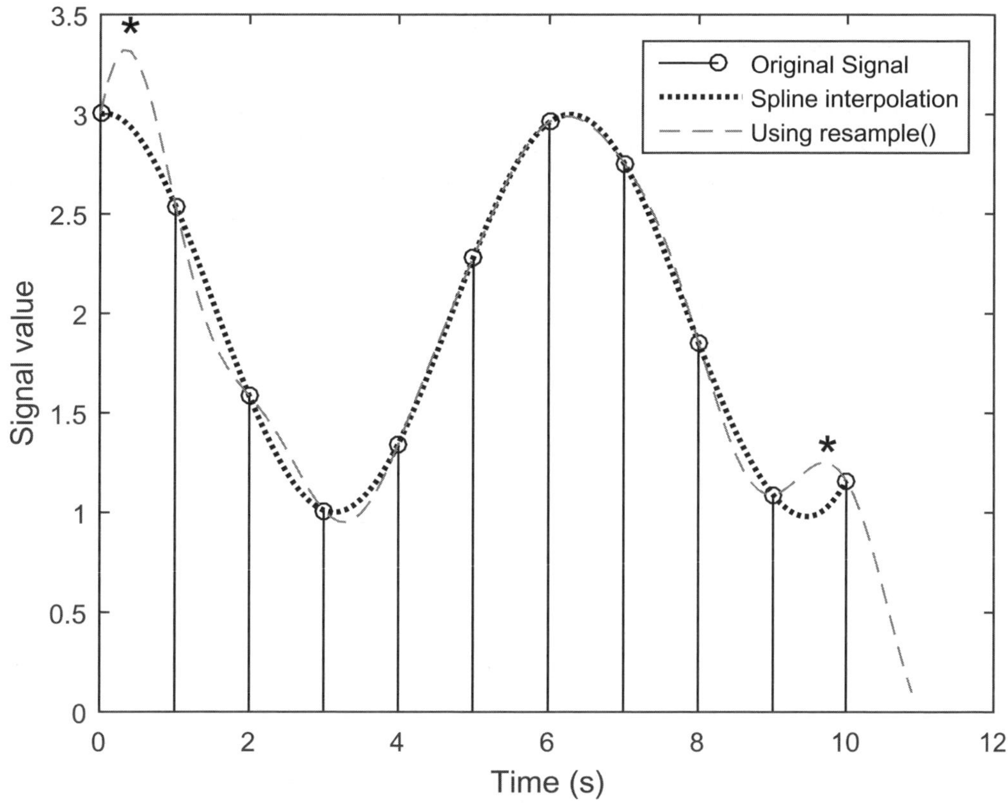

Figure 2–10. Example of spline interpolation versus resampling.

```
% Perform spline interpolation using finer time intervals.
t2 = 0:0.1:10;
y2 = spline(t, y, t2);

% Plot interpolated signal.
hold on
plot(t2, y2)

% Resample at 10x using resample() to show edge effects.
tr = (0:(length(y)-1))/10;
yr = resample(y, 10, 1);
plot(tr, yr);
```

References

Nyquist, H. (1928). Certain topics in telegraph transmission theory. *Transactions of the American Institute of Electrical Engineers*, *47*(2), 617–644.

Shannon, C. E. (1949). Communication in the presence of noise. *Proceedings of the Institute of Radio Engineers*, *37*, 10–21.

3

Interfacing With Software

Introduction

This chapter discusses interfacing MATLAB with a variety of software tools commonly used in speech, language, and hearing research. While not current in clinical practice to date, these applications are beginning to find their way into practice. Generally speaking, not only do they afford the clinician greater control over stimulus design and implementation, they also expand the range and precision of clinical intervention and assessment. In general, interfacing can be accomplished with one of three methods.

The first, and likely the easiest, involves offline processing via exchanges of files. A software package such as E-Prime (Psychology Software Tools, 2001), for example, may be used to present stimuli for a speech-production task and to record the resultant responses in a set of data files in the `.wav` format; these audio files could then be imported into MATLAB for later management, preprocessing, or analysis. In the other direction, MATLAB could be used to preprocess some signal data, and then export selected measurements from it into an Excel spreadsheet for further analysis with prewritten macros or cell formulas. For experimental setups, a researcher could use MATLAB to synthesize speech stimuli and export these as `.wav` files for playback in E-Prime or a similar stimulus presentation tool. While such file exchanges can easily be done manually, the greatest efficiency is found when their corresponding commands are incorporated into a MATLAB script, possibly using temporary files as part of a project workflow.

The second method involves using preexisting interface libraries that have been written for the environment in question. These will often "wrap" calls to functions in one language in the syntax of the other, and can interface in both directions. That is, a MATLAB user may use MATLAB code in a native `.m` file to call an external program, supply data, and obtain returned results without the need to export or import files, or a user of the external program may call MATLAB code from within it. The choice of interface direction is often dictated by the nature of the project or task. For data collection, it is often desirable to run the external environment as the master process and then call MATLAB code after recording to preprocess or analyze the data. For data visualization or interactive exploration, on the other hand, it is likely more useful to run MATLAB as the master process and write function calls out to various libraries or environments.

The third and final method we discuss requires the use of network sockets, which are software abstractions that allow one to "connect" a client process to a server process, possibly on the same machine. In this method, both environments will run simultaneously, with one making requests and receiving data from the other. In fact, many preexisting interface libraries use sockets as their underlying data flow mechanism. Due to the importance of this technology in data flow and in developing custom experimental setups, the final section of this chapter is devoted to the creation of custom server and client programs in MATLAB, which can then be modified to interface with any socket-compatible environment.

Microsoft Excel

Despite its ubiquity, Excel is not a true database management system. It allows users to enter any type of data into any cell and contains large amounts of formatting options that are not strictly necessary for data analysis. This flexibility, however, has endeared it to many in the research community, and as such, Excel is a de facto standard for data storage. Many speech and hearing data sets are likely to be in Excel format in addition to whatever proprietary or custom file formats their authors use. Furthermore, many pieces of software designed for handling data from instrumentation are likely to possess an "Export to Excel" or other similarly named feature.

As discussed in previous chapters, MATLAB includes a set of functions that can read and write Excel files for data analysis. These include `xlsread()` and `xlswrite()` and can be used flexibly through proper specification of cell arrays in input or output arguments. For `xlsread()`, the canonical output arguments are indicated in the following function call:

```
>> [num, txt, raw] = xlsread('mydata.xls');
```

The `num` output argument is a matrix including only those cells that MATLAB is able to convert into an internal numeric representation. For all other cells (e.g., text), the value of `NaN` (not a number) is used to indicate invalid numeric data. Rows of `NaN`s are excluded from this matrix. If cells containing a formula are specified, the evaluated value of the formula (if numeric) is statically included, but the formula itself will not be. As such, any changes in the original file or corresponding cells in the `num` matrix will not be reflected in the target cell.

The `txt` argument, on the other hand, contains a cell array of all text strings in the range selected, with empty strings for those values convertible into the `num` matrix. Rows of empty strings are excluded from this matrix.

If the spreadsheet of interest includes a mixture of text and numeric data, as is likely the case, it may be advisable to use the `raw` output argument. Unlike `num` and `txt`, the `raw` output cell array preserves the location of cells without removing blank rows; as such, it is useful to ensure that MATLAB "sees" the Excel data properly before doing any further conversions or processing.

In addition to the abovementioned functions, a relatively new feature of MATLAB is the `table` object. Unlike the simpler numeric or character arrays, tables can hold heterogeneous data and are especially well suited to contain research or clinical data sets. Assuming proper formatting in the source file, the following command will read an Excel spreadsheet into a MATLAB table object. Table objects are examined in greater detail in **Chapter 5**.

```
>> myTbl = readTable('myData.xls');
```

For dynamic interfacing with Excel, Spreadsheet Link™ EX can be used. This product allows access to MATLAB functionality from within Excel and does not require writing a custom import script in MATLAB. Rather, MATLAB code is executed with the `matlabfcn()` wrapper function in an Excel spreadsheet cell.

Python

The Python language, developed by van Rossum (1995), is a free, cross-platform language suited for a variety of tasks. It is often employed in quick development and prototyping and is useful for writing preprocessing scripts, especially for textual data. Furthermore, with the usage of libraries such as PsychoPy and PyGame, researchers can develop interactive stimulus presentations within Python that can collect and preprocess data before handing them off to MATLAB for the computational "heavy lifting."

A connection between MATLAB and Python can be established from either end. The `mlabwrap` library (Schmolnk & Rathod, 2011), for example, allows a Python program to call MATLAB code as though it were a normal Python library. As such, any custom scripts or analysis programs written in MATLAB can be accessed in real time from, say, a stimulus-presentation script in Python, rather than using offline processing through files.

A socket-based solution for calling MATLAB code from Python is `pymatbridge` (Jaderberg, 2011), which serves as a bridge from Python to MATLAB as its name implies. Using this bridge, a MATLAB server program is initiated on the same machine, and any function contained in a preexisting `.m` file can be executed. This interface is particularly user friendly in its use of the python dictionary type, which allows access to named input and output arguments.

The `matpy` library (Adaszewski, 2012), on the other hand, allows one to call Python code from within MATLAB. This is often helpful in expanding the plotting options available and can be used to display native MATLAB data with Python graphics libraries such as matplotlib (Hunter, 2007) and Mayavi (Ramachandran & Varoquaux, 2011). Listing 3–1 takes some sample "data," exports it to Python, runs a Python plotting script on the data, and displays the resultant graphic.

Listing 3–1. Example interface to Python via the py_eval function:

```
% Generate a random signal
x = rand(1000, 1) * 2 - 1;

% Export the data to Python using matpy.
% This will create a variable named x in the Python workspace,
% which can then be accessed by Python code.
% Note the quotes around the variable name!
py_export('x');

% Within Python, import the matplotlib library.
% This is an example of "wrapping" Python code in MATLAB syntax, and
% is only practical for short commands.
py_eval('import matplotlib as plt');

% For longer sequences of commands, it is desirable to save the
% Python script in an external file, say "tempScript.py", in the same
% folder as our .m file, then call it with a custom function built
% on py_eval().
run_pyscript('tempScript.py');
```

Listing 3–2 reproduces a custom function that calls an external Python script and runs it in the current Python session. Note that this is different from running a Python program alone, as the script can make use of variables that have been exported to the Python workspace via `py_export()`.

Listing 3–2. run_pyscript.m

```
function run_pyscript(myFile)
% Run a python script from a file using matpy.

    % Open the script for reading.
    fid = fopen(myFile, 'r');
    if (fid == -1)
        return;
    end

    % Read all lines from the script.
    % Use fgetl to keep newline characters for use in py() function
    lines = [];
    tempLine = fgets(fid);
    while ischar(tempLine)
        lines = [lines, tempLine];
        tempLine = fgets(fid);
    end

    % Close script file.
    fclose(fid);

    % Execute the script in Python.
    pyCode = sprintf(lines);
    py('eval', pyCode);
```

The (admittedly simple) Python script used in Listing 3–2 is reproduced in Listing 3–3.

Listing 3–3. tempScript.py

```
fig, (ax1, ax2) = plt.subplots(ncols=2)
ax1.plot(x)
ax1.set_title('Raw waveform')
ax2.hist(x**2, 10, histtype='stepfilled')
ax2.set_title('Histogram of squared amplitudes')
plt.show()
```

Python finds most use for the speech researcher in animation and interactive stimulus presentation rather than in data processing. While this text does not aim to teach the Python language, numerous examples exist using PyGame and PsychoPy which allow the researcher to capture experimental data in Python, then export it into MATLAB.

One particularly interesting application of Python is in the control of electroencephalogram (EEG) recordings for auditory perception experiments using EGI Net Station equipment (Electrical Geodesics, Inc., Eugene, Oregon). This uses the `pynetstation` module to send time-stamped events to the Net Station while recording user input.

Praat

Praat (Boersma & Weenik, 2001, 2014) is a well-known application designed for phonetic and acoustic analysis, with features for such tasks as spectral analysis, formant identification, pitch tracking, and glottal pulse identification, among many others. Custom analysis tasks can be automated in Praat using the Praat scripting language (e.g., the Prosogram) (Mertens, 2004).

For most features, Praat can export a text file containing the relevant information. These text files can then be imported for later analysis in MATLAB. For example, suppose we wish to track the first formant in a monosyllabic word and then do an analysis on the formant trajectory with respect to time.

For access to Praat's inbuilt capabilities from other programming languages such as MATLAB, the praatcon command-line utility is indispensable. This utility allows automated execution of preexisting Praat scripts (`.praat` files) with optional arguments, can output the result to a command window, save to a file, and so on. Here we use the MATLAB `system()` function, which submits its argument as a command to the underlying operating system.

Suppose we have a custom Praat script (say, `ap.praat`) that performs a specialized prosodic analysis on the submitted `.wav` file, but before doing the analysis we want to perform some preprocessing in MATLAB, say a low-pass filter to highlight prosodic information and remove high-frequency transients. Listing 3–4 shows one way to accomplish this programmatically.

Listing 3–4. Preprocessing in MATLAB followed by Praat analysis and MATLAB plotting

```
% Select a file for analysis.
[myFile, myPath] = uigetfile('*.wav', 'Open data file...');
```

```
% Check to make sure a file was actually selected.
if any(myPath == 0)
    return
end

% Open the wave file.
myFile = fullfile(myPath, myFile);
[y, fs] = audioread(myFile);

% Perform filtering operation(s). Here we use a 5th-order Butterworth
% filter with a cutoff frequency of 325 Hz.
cutoffFreq = 325;
filterOrder = 5;
[B, A] = butter(order, 2 * cutoffFreq / fs);
x = filter(B, A, x);

% Save the filtered signal to a temporary file.
audiowrite('temp.wav', y, fs);

% Run our custom Praat script.
% We expect the output to be a CSV file called 'temp.csv'.
system('Praatcon.exe ap.praat temp.wav')

% Load the prosodic data and plot in MATLAB.
prosodyData = csvread('temp.csv');
plot(prosodyData);
```

Note that the above script is for the Windows command line. For Linux, Unix, or Mac OS X, we would instead use the command `system('Praat ap.praat temp.wav')`.

Alternatively, we may wish to perform the preliminary steps in Praat, and then import the result into MATLAB. For example, suppose we have a large number of monosyllabic words recorded as responses to an experimental task, and we wish to determine the average voice pitch produced during each word, say for comparisons among experimental conditions or demographic factors. The following MATLAB code in Listing 3–5, using the `praatcon` command-line interface and assuming the existence of some `getpitch.praat` script, can automate this task, which might otherwise take hours of point-and-click monotony.

Listing 3–5. Using MATLAB to automate analysis in Praat

```
% Select a list of files for analysis. These can be located anywhere.
% Note: myFiles will be a cell array of strings.
[myFiles, myPath] = uigetfile('*.wav', 'Open data file...', ...
    'MultiSelect', 'on');

% Check to make sure files were actually selected.
if any(myPath == 0)
    return
end

% Preallocate a column vector for speed.
numFiles = length(myFiles);
pitches = zeros(numFiles, 1);

% Loop through list of files.
for n = 1:numFiles

    % Open the nth wave file.
    tempFile = fullfile(myPath, myFiles{n});
    [y, fs] = audioread(myFile);

    % Save to temporary file where Praatcon can access (working dir).
    audiowrite('temp.wav', y, fs);

    % Run our custom Praat script, which extracts the pitch listing.
    % We expect the output to be a CSV file called 'temp.csv'.
    system('Praatcon.exe getpitch.praat temp.wav');

    % Load the pitch data from the temporary output file.
    pitchData = csvread('temp.csv');

    % Compute mean pitch for the file. Assume that the 'getpitch'
    % script automatically excludes regions where pitch computations
    % are nonsensical, such as consonant stop gaps, frication,
    % and pauses.
    tempPitch = mean(pitchData);
```

```
    % Append result to the preallocated MATLAB column vector.
    pitches(n) = tempPitch;

end

% We now have a vector of pitches and can perform statistical or
% numerical operations on them.
mean(pitches)
std(pitches)
% etc...
```

Java

Java (Gosling & McGilton, 1995) is a programming language used on millions of devices, and it is noted for its implementation of a virtual machine across platforms. Java code, once compiled, can run on a Java virtual machine, and will in theory behave similarly regardless of the underlying hardware. In fact, MATLAB is partly based on Java for much of its functionality, particularly graphical display and networking (Altman, 2011). As such, access to Java code, classes, and packages from within MATLAB is well supported.

Java classes (`.class` files) are accessed from within MATLAB by means of the class path. This is a set of locations in which MATLAB will search for a Java class, and composes a static path loaded at startup and a dynamic path customizable within a MATLAB session. While editing the static-path config files results in faster loading, it is recommended that users new to this type of interfacing use the `javaclasspath()` function. That way, errors in programming or path specification can simply be remedied by reissuing the command without having to restart MATLAB or fix a broken config file.

Interactive Experiments With Processing

Processing (Reas & Fry, 2006) is both a Java library and a stand-alone programming environment focused on developing interactive visualizations and applications, called "sketches." An attractive feature of this environment for clinicians and researchers in speech is the relative ease with which one can create simple "testing" tasks that present targeted phonemes, words, or even practice passages while simultaneously recording the speech signal and rewarding the client with feedback through animations, graphics, or sounds.

Even though the Psychophysics Toolbox (PPT) (Brainard, 1997; Kleiner, Brainard, & Pelli, 2007; Pelli, 1997) is a well-known and reliable set of functions for stimulus presentation in MATLAB software, it can be challenging to first-time programmers to write interaction code, as all checks for mouse-clicks and key-presses must be sequenced in a main loop. If a block of code within this loop enters an infinite cycle (e.g., due to misspecification of loop limits or a simple programming mistake), it may be impossible for PPT to recover critical key-presses for cancellation. Processing sidesteps this issue through the use of multithreading, in which mouse and keyboard listeners are implemented as separate subtasks (threads) that communicate with the main thread (stimulus presentation). Typically, MATLAB does not allow user specification of separate threads but does perform multithreaded processing for linear algebra, numerical functions, and parallel computing with the Parallel Computing Toolbox.

Another pedagogical advantage of processing is the universal `exit()` method, initially wired to the ESC key. No matter how badly a prototype experiment crashes, one can always hit ESC and return to the development environment. Critically for researchers, the `exit()` method can also be overridden or expanded so that before terminating due to the user's (possibly accidental) hitting of the ESC key, the experiment can save its state to the hard drive and avoid losing the data collected to that point. This may be especially useful in experiments involving children, for example.

Depicted in Figure 3–1 is the main Processing window with several simple functions outlined. This book does not aim to be a Processing tutorial, but we note the presence of several useful, predefined functions that set up listeners for key events in experimental setups, such as key-presses and mouse-clicks. Another feature is the definition of separate `setup()` and `draw()` functions, which define the setup and looping/stimulus presentation sections of the experiment, respectively. The key-press and mouse-click listeners will call the `keyPressed()` and `mouseClicked()` functions, respectively, when a relevant event is detected, and are integral in creating interactive environments for data collection.

Because Processing is implemented as a Java class, it is possible to call Processing sketches from within MATLAB software. This approach leverages the computational power of MATLAB, while allowing researchers to develop innovative presentations in Processing.

Technically, Processing sketches are subclasses of the PApplet class, with the above-named key functions serving as methods of this subclass.

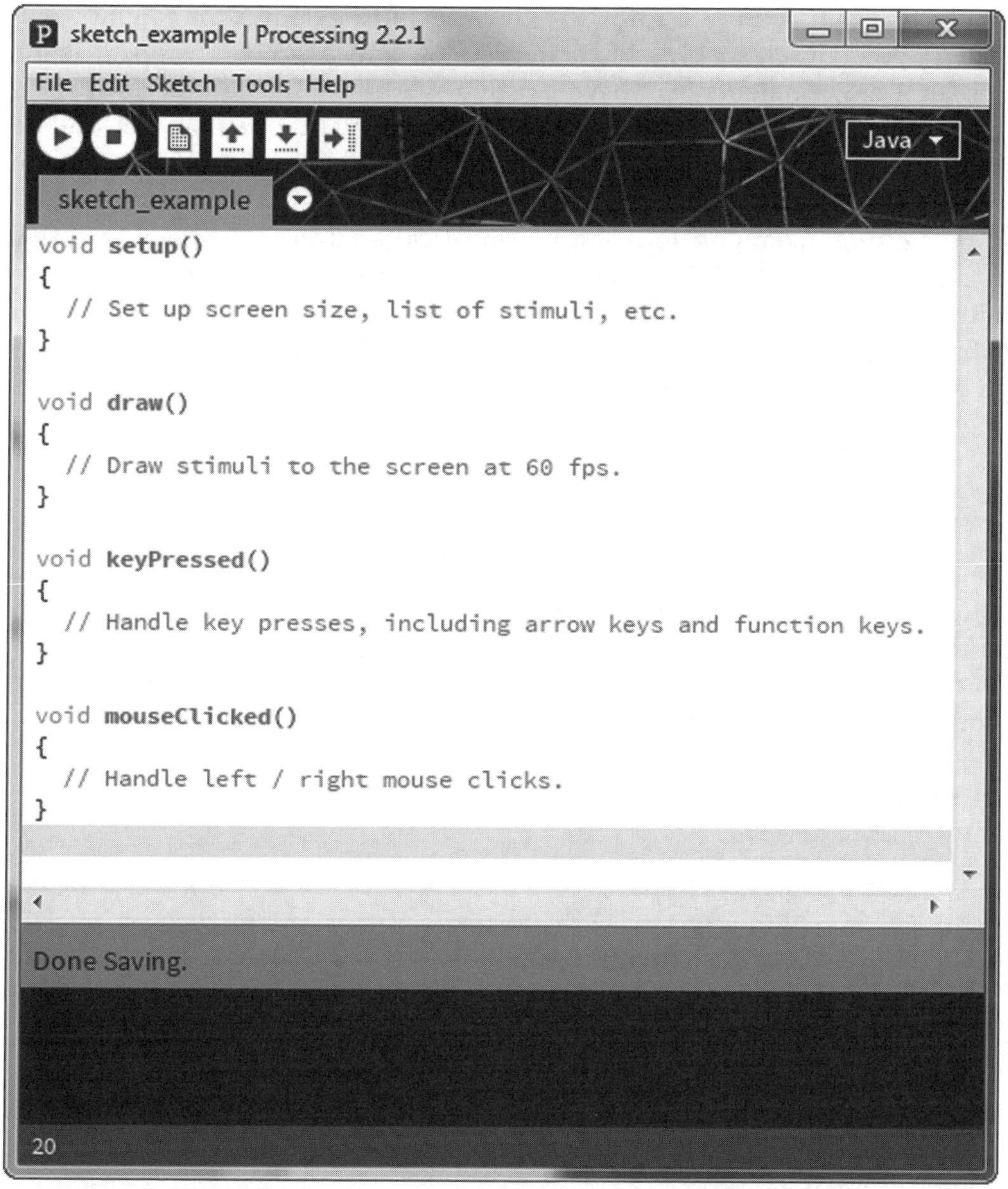

Figure 3–1. The Processing environment with several key functions indicated.

Statistical Analysis in SAS and R

As discussed previously, MATLAB software can be extended by the addition of toolboxes, or libraries of functions. One such toolbox is the Statistics

Toolbox (examined in **Chapter 5**), which includes features for common statistical procedures such as linear regression and ANOVA. However, many research environments may have existing workflows using other statistical or graphical programs such as SAS, SPSS, and R. This section will outline steps useful in exporting MATLAB data into file formats readable by common statistical software.

The most common formats for statistical analysis are generally Excel (`.xls`, `.xlsx`) or CSV (comma-separated value, `.csv`). These can contain mixed numeric and character data, and therefore require use of cell arrays or tables to appropriately combine the various data types. Data export proceeds in two steps: (a) constructing a combined table or cell array and (b) performing file operations.

Constructing a Cell Array From an Existing Data Set

Regardless of the number of variables involved, the end goal of this step is a single cell array, possibly with a first row of headers. If the data are already entirely numeric and in a single matrix, then the process is relatively simple. In the example below, suppose we have a matrix `M` with three numeric columns, and we wish to export them under the names X, Y, and Z:

```
% Transform matrix into a cell array.
data = num2cell(M);

% Add headers (optional).
headers = {'X', 'Y', 'Z'};
data = vertcat(headers, data);
```

The first block converts the matrix to a cell array, whereas the second appends a row of headers. In the case where we have separate variables, they must first be horizontally concatenated. This can be accomplished as follows. Suppose we have the numeric column vectors `ID`, `Stimulus`, and `ResponseTime`:

```
% Combine data into a single matrix.
M = [ID, Stimulus, ResponseTime];

% Transform matrix into a cell array.
data = num2cell(M);

% Add headers (optional).
headers = {'Patient ID', 'Stimulus Code', 'Response Time'};
data = vertcat(headers, data);
```

If we have separate MATLAB variables with different types, these must first be converted to cell arrays before concatenation. Suppose that, in the following example, the variable `ID` contains multiple-character strings such as `'0145'`, `'101b'`, and so forth, and is already a cell array:

```
% Convert remaining variables to cell arrays.
Stimulus = num2cell(Stimulus);
ResponseTime = num2cell(ResponseTime);

% Combine data into a single matrix.
M = [ID, Stimulus, ResponseTime];

% Transform matrix into a cell array.
data = num2cell(M);

% Add headers (optional).
headers = {'Patient ID', 'Stimulus Code', 'Response Time'};
data = vertcat(headers, data);
```

The first block of code converts each variable to its own cell array. Because all variables now have the same type (cell), they can be easily concatenated using standard matrix notation. The remainder of the program functions identically as in the previous examples.

File Operations

Now that the MATLAB-generated data are packaged for export, we instruct our program to save them to a standard file format for interoperability. Despite the utility and flexibility of `.mat` files, it is advisable to save into Excel or CSV formats as most statistical software cannot access data inside a `.mat` file. This can be done using the `xlswrite()` function, which supports `.xlsx`, `.xlsb`, `.xlsm`, and `.xls` formats. Note the use of the `fullfile()` function for cross-platform path-string compatibility:

```
% Select where to save the file.
[myOutputFile, myPath] = uiputfile('*.xlsx', 'Export to Excel...');

% Check if a proper location was selected.
if any(myPath == 0)
    return
end

% Construct the full path to the output file.
myOutputFile = fullfile(myPath, myOutputFile);
```

```
% Export the data to the selected file.
xlswrite(myOutputFile, data);
```

Sockets and Networking

Many of the above-named toolboxes and routines are built on top of a socket implementation in MATLAB. This allows MATLAB to act as a server and receive data from external programs in real time. This section outlines the creation and usage of socket-based server and client programs for data transfer in MATLAB.

Setting Up a Server

Probably the most straightforward way of creating a server in MATLAB is through the Instrument Control Toolbox, a set of routines designed for connection to a variety of hardware instruments. However, the functions are not limited to hardware but also allow communication with running software tools as virtual instruments, as it were.

A server is created with the `tcpip()` function, which uses the TCP/IP interface to listen for remote connections. A typical server-initiation call is below. For this example, we use the port number 12345; however, any port number can be used as long as it does not conflict with common services. For this purpose, high port numbers are recommended:

```
% Create a server.
myServer = tcpip('localhost', 12345, 'NetworkRole', 'server');

% Listen for incoming connection.
fopen(myServer);
```

Readers may notice the similarity of the `fopen` function to that used in Chapter 1 to handle binary data. An important aspect of this usage of `fopen` is that the function will not return (i.e., pass control back to the calling scope) until an incoming connection is received. Once the `fopen` command is completed, data can be read from the stream using `fread`. We use the `BytesAvailable` property of the `myServer` object to ensure that we read the correct amount of bytes:

```
myData = fread(myServer, myServer.BytesAvailable);
```

At this point, the data have been successfully transferred to the variable `myData`, and can be analyzed, plotted, filtered, or saved to the host computer.

Using MATLAB® as a Client

In some cases, we might wish to send data from MATLAB to an external program acting as a server. The code is remarkably similar to the above. We first create an outgoing socket interface by using the `tcpip` function, but this time we set the `NetworkRole` property to `'client'`:

```
myClient = tcpip('localhost', 12345, 'NetworkRole', 'client');
```

We then open the connection and send the data, which are stored in the variable `myData` for the purposes of this example:

```
% Open the connection to the server.
fopen(myClient);

% Send data.

fwrite(myClient, myData);
```

References

Adaszewski, S. (2012). matpy [computer software]. Retrieved from http://algoholic.eu/matpy/

Altman, Y. (2011). *Undocumented secrets of MATLAB®-Java programming*. Boca Raton, FL: CRC Press.

Boersma, P., & Weenik, D. (2001). Praat, a system for doing phonetics by computer. *Glot International*, *5*(9/10), 341–345.

Boersma, P., & Weenik, D. (2014). Praat: Doing phonetics by computer [Computer program]. Version 5.3.84. Retrieved August 26, 2014, from http://www.praat.org/

Brainard, D. H. (1997). The Psychophysics Toolbox. *Spatial Vision*, *10*, 433–436.

Gosling, J., & McGilton, H. (1995). *The Java language environment: A white paper*. Mountain View, CA: Sun Microsystems.

Hunter, J. D. (2007). matplotlib [computer software]. Retrieved from http://matplotlib.org/

Jaderberg, M. (2011). Python-Matlab-bridge v0.5.2-18 [Computer software]. Retrieved from http://arokem.github.io/python-matlab-bridge/

Kleiner, M., Brainard, D., & Pelli, D. (2007). What's new in Psychtoolbox-3? *Perception*, *36*, ECVP Abstract Supplement.

Mertens, P. (2004). Un outil pour la transcription de la prosodie dans les corpus oraux [A tool for transcription of prosody in speech corpora]. *Traitement Automatique des Langues*, *45*(2), 109–130.

Pelli, D. G. (1997). The VideoToolbox software for visual psychophysics: Transforming numbers into movies. *Spatial Vision*, *10*, 437–442.

Ramachandran, P., & Varoquaux, G. (2011). Mayavi: 3D visualization of scientific data. *Computing in Science & Engineering, 13*(2), 40–51.

Reas, C., & Fry, B. (2006). Processing: Programming for the media arts. *AI & Society, 20*(4), 526–538.

Schmolck, A., & Rathod, V. (2011). Mlabwrap v1.1 [Computer software]. Retrieved from http://mlabwrap.sourceforge.net/

Van Rossum, G. (1995). Python tutorial. *Centrum voor Wiskunde en Informatica Technical Report*, CI-R9526.

4

Applications of MATLAB® in Clinical and Research Settings

Stimulus Generation and Presentation

Before a test can be given, a sound file played, or a response item assessed, one must first have the item in question created, stored, and prepared for presentation. This section covers the generation of auditory stimuli *ex nihilo* (i.e., by synthesis) as well as the modification of existing speech data for this purpose. We begin with a basic treatment of sinewave synthesis and then cover three modes of speech synthesis: the classic Klatt synthesizer, articulatory synthesis as informed by the increasingly popular DIVA model, and sinewave speech.

Sinewave Synthesis

As a stimulus, sine tones are most pervasive in hearing practice. Audiograms, for example, are obtained by testing a patient's response to a series of sine tones at different frequencies and intensities. Although the use of sine tones in speech practice is more limited, useful applications nonetheless include cueing, as in emulating notes in intonation and rhythm exercises, or in auditory feedback.

In MATLAB, a researcher or clinician can create and present sine tones with a handful of commands. Listing 4–1 demonstrates the production of a one-second, 440-Hz sine tone at a sampling rate of 10 kHz. Note that we use the `sound()` function as opposed to `soundsc()` in order to preserve the relative amplitude.

Listing 4–1. Synthesis and presentation of a 440-Hz sinewave

```
% Define sampling rate and frequency of interest.
fs = 10000;
freq = 440;

% Create time vector.
time = (1:fs) / fs;

% Synthesize a sine tone.
y = sin(2*pi*freq*time);

% Play back.
sound(y, fs)
```

Drawing on the concept of a function discussed earlier, we may abstract this technique into a modular function stored in a `.m` file. Listing 4–2 contains code for such a function, which accepts frequency, amplitude, and duration as parameters. Note that the latter two arguments are optional, and we test for their inclusion using the special `nargin` function.

Listing 4–2. A function to play sine tones of arbitrary frequency, intensity, and duration

```
function playsine(freq, amp, duration)
% PLAYSINE Play sine tone at specified frequency, amplitude, and duration.
% PLAYSINE(440, 1) plays a 440-Hz tone at max amplitude for 1 second.
% PLAYSINE(1000, 0.5, 0.25) plays a 1000-Hz tone at half amplitude for a
% duration of 250 milliseconds.

    % Use CD-audio standard sampling rate.
    fs = 44100;
```

```
    % Check for duration.
    if nargin < 3
        duration = 1;
    end

    % Create time vector based on duration.
    time = (1:fs*duration) / fs;

    % Check for amplitude.
    if nargin < 2
       amp = 1;
    else
       % Ensure supplied amplitude is positive and does not exceed 1.
       amp = min(abs(amp), 1);
    end

    % Synthesize sine wave.
    y = amp * sin(2*pi*freq*time);

    % Play back.
    sound(y, fs)

end
```

Assuming a calibrated set of headphones and a table corresponding floating-point amplitude values to intensities in decibel sound pressure level (dB_{SPL}), the above code would be sufficient to run a simple audiogram, or even to test overall hearing range regardless of acuity. One practical and entertaining classroom exercise involves determining the maximum hearing frequency of the student body.

Exercises

1. Why do we include the factor of `2*pi` in the `sin()` function?
2. What would happen if we allowed the amplitude to exceed 1? Recall the common limitations on range in most sound cards and `.wav` files.
3. Rewrite the above function to return the variable `y` as a column vector (e.g., for further processing).
4. Create a function to play the same tone at increasing amplitudes, querying the user each time as to whether the tone was heard. This function

should return the amplitude at which the user indicated he or she first heard the tone. *Hint:* Use a *for* loop with the set of amplitudes 0.1, 0.2, …, 1.0. Be careful to ensure the maximum amplitude does not cause hearing damage given your audio setup.

5. Building from Exercise 3, write a function to produce a complex sine tone. The function should take the following arguments: (a) a vector of frequencies, (b) a second vector of amplitudes, and (c) duration in seconds. Ensure this function also scales the amplitude of the final wave within the ±1 limit.
6. Using nested *for* loops or any another automation technique, use Exercise 4 to produce a simple audiometer-like test setup that iterates over the standard ranges of frequencies tested (125 Hz, 250 Hz, 500 Hz, 1000 Hz, 2000 Hz, 3000 Hz, 4000 Hz, and 8000 Hz), determining the minimum amplitude at which the user can hear each tone. Plot the curve of amplitudes by tones. How is this similar to an audiogram? How does it differ? How might we improve it? As in Exercise 2, ensure your audio setup does not exceed reasonable levels even at the max amplitude of 1.

Klatt Synthesis

Even though sine tones can be reproduced or analyzed with ease, speech synthesis remains a challenge. This is because natural connected speech is highly dynamic and contains prosodic variations that are difficult to model. Even so, speech stimuli that can be useful in speech, language and hearing practice can be synthesized by means of a Klatt synthesizer (Klatt, 1980). This synthesizer is formant based, as opposed to concatenative synthesis, which pieces together prerecorded speech segments. Formants (Fant, 1960) are the resonant frequencies of the vocal tract, and vary over time as the position of the articulators changes.

The Klatt synthesizer accepts as input a set of vectors indicating the values of certain acoustic parameters over time. In particular, the vectors indicating formant frequencies, denoted F1–F6, and bandwidths are critical in producing voiced sounds, whereas the vector indicating the presence or absence of voicing allows for the specification of voiceless sounds.

Key parameters for the Klatt synthesizer derive from the source-filter model of speech, in which a sound source (voicing from the glottis, or frication/noise from a constriction) is filtered by the resonances of the vocal tract (i.e., formants) (Fant, 1960). A mixture of voicing and noise can also be produced, to synthesize voiced fricatives, for example. The glottal source is passed to the filter defined by parameters NP (nasal poles), NZ (nasal zeros), and F1–F4 (formants). F2–F6 receive the noise or friction source in parallel. The degree to which a sound is voiced depends on the mixture of AV (amplitude of voicing), AVS (amplitude of quasi-sinusoidal voicing), and AF (amplitude of frication), among several others (Klatt, 1980). Creation of nasal consonants relies on use of NP and NZ. Stops can be created by manipulating AV, AF, and AH (amplitude of aspiration).

McLennan (2000) outlines a compact Klatt synthesizer interface (http://www.shaav.com/professional/linguistics/klatt.html) in the Simulink environment, which can be automated from the Command Window. In this realization, a subset of vocal-tract parameters are generated using the `makeutt()` function and stored as a set of variables in the main Workspace. These variables are named according to the convention in Klatt (1980), facilitating direct comparison and/or modification as needed. Synthesis then proceeds by calling the `sim()` function on the `klatt.mdl` model file provided with the implementation. Listing 4–3 demonstrates the synthesis of the word "MATLAB" using the phonetic coding indicated in McLennan (2000), and adjusting the Simulink running time programmatically. The usage of `'A'` in the string `'mAtlAb'`, for example, indicates the phoneme /æ/. Note that some loading time may be necessary if Simulink has not been previously initialized.

Listing 4–3. Klatt synthesis via Simulink (McLennan, 2000)

```
% Load Klatt synthesizer model (McLennan, 2000).
load_system('klatt.mdl')

% Define utterance of interest.
u = 'mAtlAb';

% Assign vocal-tract parameters.
[F0, ttf, A2, A3, A4, A5, A6, AB, AV, AH, AF, AVS, tt, F, BW] = makeutt(u);

% Compute total simulation time with end buffer to ensure enough room for
% the final phoneme. Generally 1000 ms is sufficient.
% Note that the stop time must be specified as a string.
totalTime = tt(end) + 1000;
stopTime = num2str(totalTime);

% Run simulation.
s = sim('klatt.mdl', 'StopTime', stopTime);
```

```
% Extract and scale output.
y = get(s, 'utterance');
y = y / max(y);

% Plot with proper timescale.
fs = 10000;
time = (1:length(y)) / fs;
plot(time, y)
xlabel('Time (s)')
ylabel('Y')
ylim([-1, 1])

% Play sound.
sound(y, fs)
```

Exercises

1. What would happen if we changed the sampling rate in the above code without modifying the original simulation files?
2. How does formant synthesis differ from other techniques, such as concatenative synthesis?
3. Using the above code as a template, create a function that accepts a phonetic string as input and outputs the synthesized signal. Be sure to use proper assignment statements to place the outputs of `makeutt()` in the Workspace.

Sinewave Speech Synthesis

In contrast to Klatt synthesis, sinewave speech synthesis (e.g., Remez et al., 1981; Rubin, 1980) proceeds by generating pure sine tones at the frequencies specified by the formant tracks. It is used, among other things, for investigating the nature of speech perception versus general auditory perception. Although it has relatively poor quality in and of itself, its perceptibility is striking in the total absence of other speech cues. Specifically, speech produced from sinewave synthesis lacks the harmonics produced in human speech from glottal vibrations; as such, this speech cannot be said to contain a "real" voice as commonly defined, leading to some difficulties in replicating voiceless consonants.

Sinewave speech synthesis (SWS) can proceed purely from a set of parameters, or can be a resynthesis of an existing speech sample. We will examine the second approach, which uses a set of MATLAB routines (Ellis,

2004) to extract parameters from a user-specified audio file and then feeds the parameters into the Haskins Laboratory MATLAB functions (Rubin, Ellis, & Frost, 1996; see http://www.haskins.yale.edu/featured/sws/MATLAB/matlab.html) to produce audio data. Listing 4–4 imports an audio file of the user's choosing, extracts the SWS parameters, then produces and plays a SWS signal. For simplicity, it is assumed that the user selects a valid `.wav` file.

Listing 4–4. Function for sinewave speech resynthesis

```
function swsfromfile()
% SWSFROMFILE Perform sine-wave speech resynthesis from a .wav file.

    % Get file from UI selector.
    [fileName, filePath] = uigetfile('*.wav', 'Select source file...');
    fileName = fullfile(filePath, fileName);

    % Import audio.
    [y, fs] = audioread(fileName);

    % Extract SWS parameters.
    [freqs, magnitudes] = swsmodel(y, fs);

    % Resynthesize and play.
    y2 = synthtrax(freqs, magnitudes, fs);
    sound(y2, fs)
end
```

Exercises

1. How does sinewave speech synthesis differ from formant synthesis?
2. What would happen if the output variable magnitudes were multiplied by some constant? Try plotting the transpose of magnitudes and comparing it to the original signal.
3. Create a function using the above code, but restrict synthesis to components below a specified cutoff frequency. Hint: Use logical indexing on the freqs vector.
4. The result of the `swsmodel()` function can be "jumpy." Apply a smoothing algorithm (such as moving-window averaging; see **Chapter 2**) before resynthesis and observe the changes in the result.
5. Using GUIDE, design a graphical user interface (GUI) for sinewave synthesis and plotting. You may use any of the standard MATLAB UI

functions. The GUI should contain two axes objects for side-by-side comparisons of the original and resynthesized signal.

6. Write a script that combines the Klatt interface functionality (McLennan, 2000) with sinewave speech synthesis. Specifically, determine which output argument(s) correspond to formant frequencies and amplitudes, and then modify these vectors to work with the `synthtrax()` function. Remember that the Klatt interface uses a sampling frequency of 10 kHz.

Articulatory Speech Synthesis Informed by the DIVA Model

The DIVA model (Directions into Velocities of Articulators; Guenther, 1994; Guenther, Ghosh, & Tourville, 2006) is a widely accepted model of speech production that, unlike the Klatt synthesizer, is articulator based. This model was developed with the intent to synthesize speech from a neurologically inspired series of activations in the vocal tract, and has in fact served as the foundation for developing a neural decoder used to allow persons with locked-in syndrome to communicate via rudimentary speech sounds via Klatt synthesis (Guenther et al., 2009).

Although not a synthesizer in itself, the DIVA model can be used to inform the generation of parameters for articulatory synthesizers. In particular, the Maeda synthesizer (e.g., Maeda, 1988) can be controlled by parameters extracted from a learning session under the DIVA framework. This synthesizer can be downloaded from http://www.cns.bu.edu/~speech/VTCalcs.php for experimentation and simulation independent of the DIVA model.

As opposed to simply accepting a list of parameters, the DIVA model aims to generate the articulatory parameters on its own through a learning procedure, where the model attempts to reach a specified acoustic target. Therefore, it is advisable to allow for multiple repetitions so that the model can better approximate the desired output.

This model accounts for a large proportion of the productive side of the speech chain. It can also be used to synthesize stimuli according to a set of model parameters, and has been implemented in the Simulink environment. As of this writing, source code is available at http://www.bu.edu/speechlab/software/diva-source-code/. The model is installed by downloading the source code and placing it in a folder to which MATLAB has access. The simple MATLAB commands in Listing 4–5 will then open the model and launch an interactive GUI for setting simulation parameters.

Listing 4–5. MATLAB® commands to initiate the DIVA GUI

```
% Open the DIVA model in Simulink.
open diva

% Launch the GUI.
diva_gui
```

In Figure 4–1, the lower-left combo box contains example productions to test the simulation. Select an appropriate example and hit "Start" to iterate over the indicated number of learning cycles.

An extension of this model is the gradient-order DIVA model (GODIVA; Bohland, Bullock, & Guenther, 2010). GODIVA aims to model the planning and execution of syllable sequences through the solution of a system of differential equations that simulate changes in certain neuron populations. Unfortunately, as of this writing, MATLAB code for the GODIVA model is not publically available.

Filtering Speech

Broadly speaking, filtering speech involves selecting or accepting a certain range of frequencies, while removing other frequencies from the signal. Filters can be broken into four types, depending on the way they handle their cutoff frequencies. Low-pass filters will remove every component above the cutoff frequency. High-pass filters, on the other hand, will keep everything above the cutoff but remove everything else. Band-pass filters will preserve frequencies between their two cutoffs, whereas notch or band-stop filters will remove them. A common use of notch filters is to remove the fundamental from a voiced signal while keeping its harmonics. In sensitive audio applications, notch filters are also used to remove line noise introduced from power outlets (60 Hz in the United States).

In addition to its ability to remove some types of noise from a speech signal, filtering can be used in the experimental domain to focus on specific aspects of speech or prosody. A low-pass filter, for example, can be used to remove the (relatively) higher-frequency components that indicate vowel or phoneme identity while preserving the fundamental frequency. In Lindfield, Wingfield, and Goodglass (1999), a cutoff frequency of 325 Hz was used to preserve the terminal word form in the prosodic domain without providing phonological information.

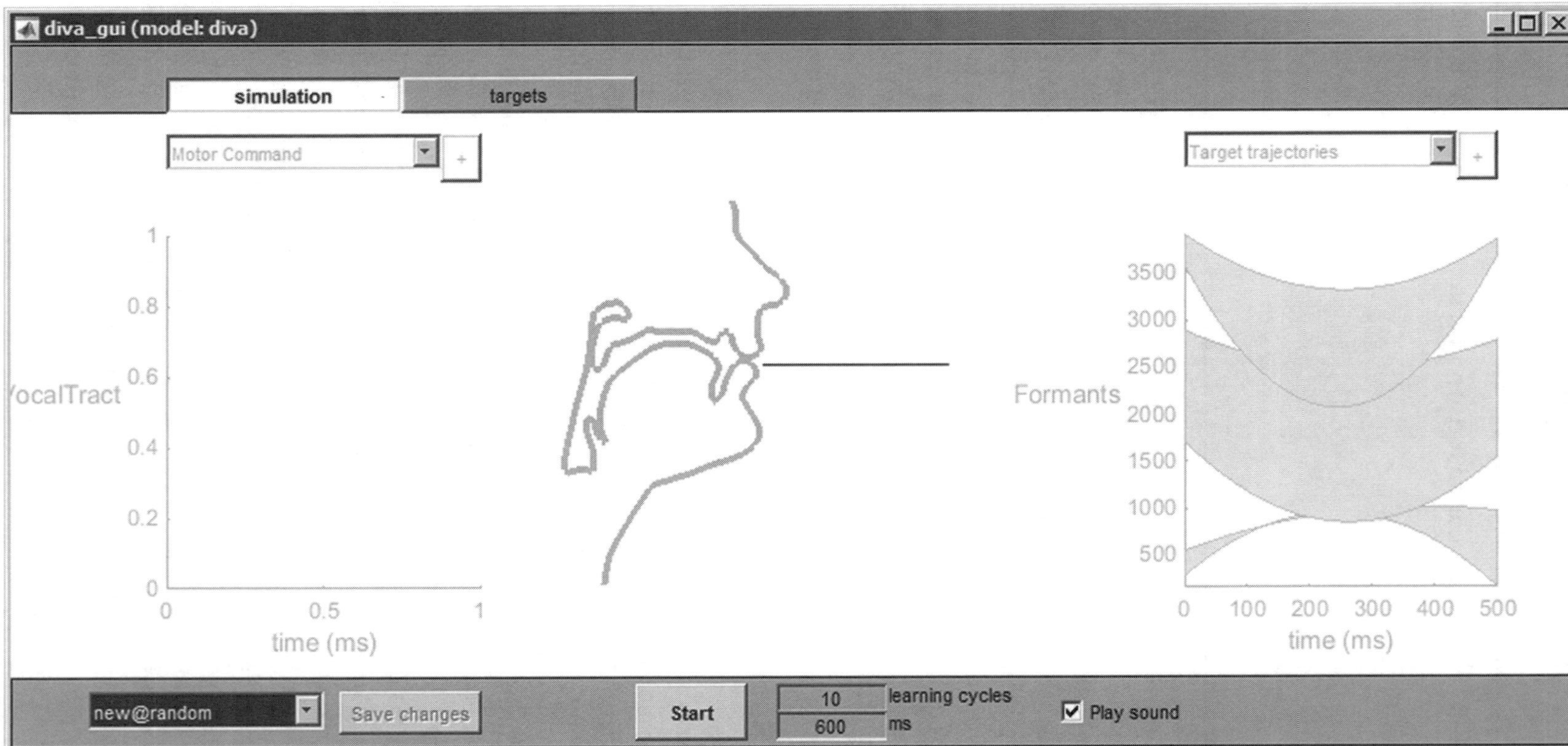

Figure 4–1. The DIVA interface.

Here we demonstrate the design and application of a Butterworth filter, which has the desirable property of preserving the frequency distribution in its pass-band (Butterworth, 1930). Listing 4–6 requires the Signal Processing Toolbox.

Listing 4–6. Application of a low-pass Butterworth filter at 325 Hz

```
function yf = lpexample(y, fs)
% LPEXAMPLE Applies a 325-Hz lowpass filter to y, sampled at fs.

    % Compute Nyquist frequency from sampling rate.
    fN = fs / 2;

    % Define cutoff frequency and compute normalized angular freq.
    cutoff = 325;
    Wn = cutoff / fN;

    % Get 6th-order filter coefficients.
    % Increase order for sharper roll-off.
    [B, A] = butter(6, Wn);

    % Plot the filter response.
    fvtool(B, A);

    % Apply filter to a signal.
    yf = filter(B, A, y);

end
```

Another way of designing filters in MATLAB involves the use of the `designfilt()` function. This function accepts a number of arguments in parameter-value pairs, and will select an appropriate filter design automatically based on the specifications. If a critical specification is missing, it will also launch a GUI and allow the user to select the appropriate parameters. The filter will be stored in a `digitalFilter` object, which can then be passed into a variety of visualization and filtering tools. This spares the user from dealing with the more technical aspects of filter coefficients, zeros, and poles.

As an example, suppose we wish to design a high-pass filter for a signal sampled at 10000 Hz, with a cutoff frequency of 300 Hz (Figure 4–2). Such a filter might be used, for example, when pre-emphasizing the higher range of frequencies prior to formant detection. In Listing 4–7, assume our signal

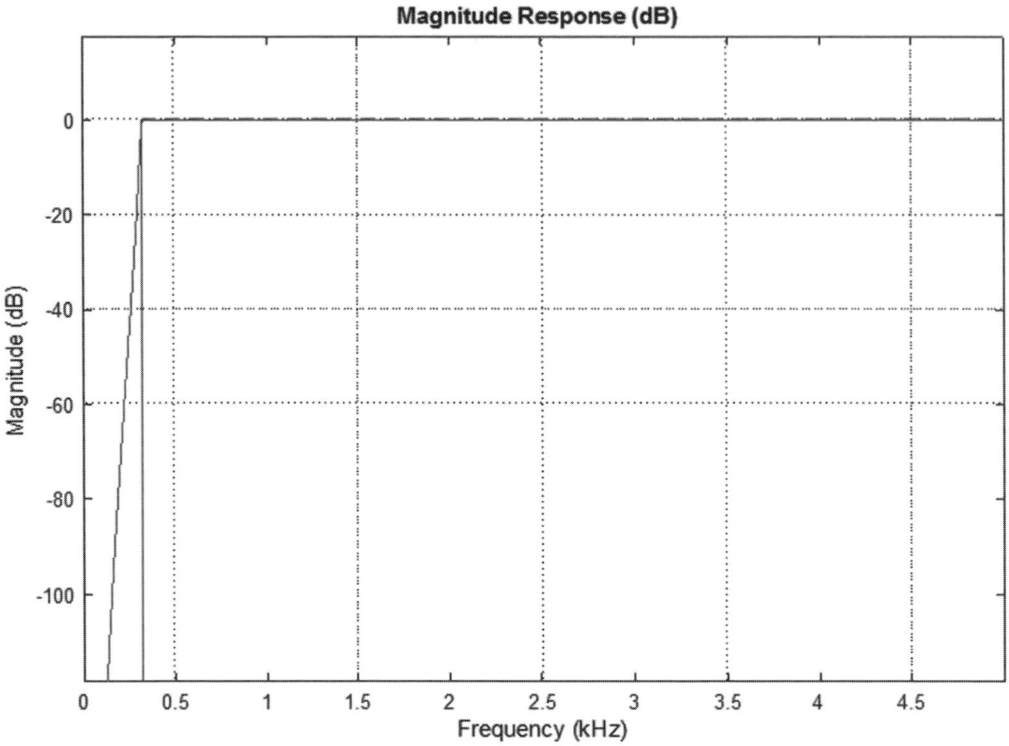

Figure 4–2. Magnitude response for a 325-Hz high-pass filter.

is saved in the variable `y`, with its sampling frequency in `fs`. We first design the filter and then visualize its response with the `fvtool()` function. We then apply the `filter()` function as above, but with a different set of arguments.

Listing 4–7. Digital filter design and application

```
% Design a high-pass filter with cutoff at 325 Hz.
f = designfilt('highpassiir', ...
    'FilterOrder', 10, ...
    'PassbandFrequency', 325, ...
    'SampleRate', fs, ...
    'PassbandRipple', 0.1);

% View the filter's response to ensure it is acceptable.
fvtool(f)

% Filter the data.
yf = filter(f, y);
```

Exercises

1. Explain the four types of filters in terms of which frequencies they pass through and which they reject or attenuate.
2. Create a band-pass filter to capture frequencies in the region of 200 to 1000 Hz.

Speech in Noise

The speech-in-noise (SIN) paradigm has been used to measure robustness of speech and hearing, particularly in the fields of audiology and bilingualism. Because noise can pose a challenge for persons with hearing loss, the SIN paradigm has been recommended for use in hearing screenings (Beck & Nilsson, 2013), heading-aid fittings (Nilsson, Soli, & Sullivan, 1994) and training programs (e.g., Song, Skoe, Banai, & Kraus, 2012). Furthermore, a growing body of research (e.g., Hervais-Adelman, Pefkou, & Golestani, 2014) has demonstrated the effect of language experience on perceptual acuity in noise. For example, as speakers gain proficiency in their second language, their ability to process their native language in noise may decrease (von Hapsburg & Bahng, 2009).

Addition of noise to a signal is easily accomplished in MATLAB. We begin with the generation of uniform white noise to achieve a specified SNR (signal-to-noise ratio) in decibels, assuming a clean source speech signal. The SNR is defined as the ratio of squared signal amplitude and the squared noise amplitude, where amplitudes are computed as RMS (not peak-to-peak). Mathematically, we write

$$SNR = \frac{A_{sig}^2}{A_{noise}^2} = \frac{RMS(y)^2}{RMS(noise)^2}$$

To express SNR in decibels, a logarithmic conversion is necessary. By the properties of logarithms, the following relationship can be obtained:

$$SNR_{dB} = 10\log_{10}(SNR)$$

$$= 10\log_{10}\left(\frac{RMS(y)^2}{RMS(noise)^2}\right)$$

$$= 20\log_{10}\left(\frac{RMS(y)}{RMS(noise)}\right)$$

By solving for the RMS of the noise signal in terms of the desired SNR in decibels, we achieve the following:

$$SNR_{dB} = 20\log_{10}\left(\frac{RMS(y)}{RMS(noise)}\right)$$

$$\frac{SNR_{dB}}{20} = \log_{10}\left(\frac{RMS(y)}{RMS(noise)}\right) = -\log_{10}\left(\frac{RMS(noise)}{RMS(y)}\right)$$

$$10^{\frac{-SNR_{dB}}{20}} RMS(y) = RMS(noise)$$

The function in Listing 4–8 opens a specified monaural audio file and then returns it with the added noise. The above equation is converted into MATLAB syntax to solve for the required noise RMS to achieve the specified SNR.

Listing 4–8. Function to add noise to a speech file

```
function y = addnoise(fileName, desiredSNR)

    % Load file.
    y = audioread(fileName);

    % Compute RMS amplitude.
    Ay = rms(y);

    % Solve for desired RMS of noise.
    An = Ay*10^-(desiredSNR / 20);

    % Generate uniform white noise.
    n = rand(size(y))*2 - 1;

    % Scale noise to achieve the desired SNR.
    n = An*n;

    % Add noise to the signal.
    y = y + n;

end
```

A similar approach can be taken with other noise types, such as conversational noise or background music. Instead of using a synthesized white noise source, one can simply import a monaural noise file and adjust its amplitude to achieve the desired SNR. The function in Listing 4–9 does just that, assuming equal sampling rates and lengths for the noise and speech files. The case of different sampling rates and/or lengths is left as an exercise for the reader.

Listing 4–9. Function to add one file as noise to a second

```
function y = addnoisefile(speechFile, noiseFile, desiredSNR)

    % Load speech file and compute amplitude.
    ySpeech = audioread(speechFile);
    ampSpeech = rms(ySpeech);

    % Load noise file and compute amplitude.
    yNoise = audioread(noiseFile);
    ampNoise = rms(yNoise);

    % Solve for desired RMS of noise and apply.
    desiredAmpNoise = ampSpeech*10^-(desiredSNR / 20);
    yNoise = yNoise * desiredAmpNoise / ampNoise;

    % Add noise to the signal.
    y = ySpeech + yNoise;

end
```

Exercises

1. Using properties of logarithms, express the SNR in decibels as a ratio of RMS amplitudes.
2. Combine the above two programs to form a generalized function that optionally accepts three versus two arguments. If three arguments are provided, use the third one as the noise file name. If only two are provided, the function should synthesize uniform white noise instead.
3. These programs assume the noise file and the target speech file have the same sampling rate, which is not always the case. Using the `resample()` function from the Signal Processing Toolbox, rewrite the programs to ensure that the noise file matches the speech file's sampling rate before combining them.
4. Expand the generalized function to include an optional fourth argument for onset time in milliseconds. The noise should be added at this onset time, rather than from the start of the speech signal. Be sure to account

for differing signal lengths, using only that portion of the noise signal corresponding to the remainder of the speech signal after the onset time.

5. It is often of interest to create dichotic stimuli (i.e., stimuli with different speech vs. noise profiles presented to each ear). Create a function that can handle stereo speech files as well as stereo noise files.

Gated Speech

The gating paradigm, first developed by Grosjean (1980), has widespread use in investigations of speech recognition and auditory perception. In this paradigm, words or stimuli are presented in a sequence of increasing "gates," and participants are tasked with recognizing the word based on this partial information. These gates may be arbitrary numbers but are usually constructed to increase in fixed increments (e.g., 50 ms). In such a scenario, the initial presentation for a given word will contain the first 50 ms of that word. Successive presentations will contain 100 ms, 150 ms, 200 ms, and so on, until the entire word is presented and/or the participant correctly guesses the word.

Constructing stimuli for such a task can be a time-consuming process, even with modern wave-editing software. The process of pointing, clicking, dragging, and selecting successively larger gate sizes is quite repetitive, and therefore highly amenable to automation in MATLAB. This section outlines the development of a gated stimulus generation program useful in a variety of laboratory or clinical settings. We also highlight the utility of abstraction, a term used in programming to refer to the practice breaking down a complex program into components that are modularized and reused.

At the lowest level, the software will need to accept a vector of audio data along with a sampling rate, select the appropriate number of samples from the onset, and return the result. For simplicity, we assume that the stimulus files have already been cleaned up to contain only the word of interest, and do not contain carrier phrases or silences around the word. Later we will explore methods of automatically detecting speech versus silence. See Listing 4–10.

Listing 4–10. Function to produce a single gated stimulus

```
function y = clipgate(y, fs, gate_ms)
% CLIPGATE Select the appropriate gated stimulus region

    % Determine the number of samples needed.
    gate_samples = round(gate_ms * fs / 1000);
```

```
    % Ensure that the selected gate size is within the signal region.
    gate_samples = max(gate_samples, 1);
    gate_samples = min(gate_samples, length(y));

    % Select the desired gate from y.
    % Note that we use matrix indexing to select all columns. This
    % accounts for stereo or multi-channel audio as well as mono.
    y = y(1:gate_samples, :);

end
```

We now turn to the process of automating the generation of gated stimuli from a single word. In Listing 4–11 we make use of the `uigetfile()` function to allow a user to select a file from a graphical window, and also demonstrate the use of optional arguments with parameter/value pairs. Furthermore, the `fileparts()` and `fullfile()` functions are used for cross-platform compatibility in generating file names for the resultant stimuli. In later programs, we will call this function with a prespecified file name.

Listing 4–11. Function to produce a sequence of gated stimuli

```
function allgates(varargin)
% ALLGATES Generate a set of gated stimuli from a .wav file.

    % Process input arguments.
    p = inputParser();
    p.addParameter('fileName', '');
    p.addParameter('gateSize', 50);
    p.parse(varargin{:});
    fileName = p.Results.fileName;
    gateSize = p.Results.gateSize;

    % If no filename is provided, prompt user for one.
    if isempty(fileName)
        [fileName, filePath] = uigetfile('*.wav', 'Open stimulus file...');

        % Check that a file was selected.
        if isempty(fileName)
            return
        end
```

```
        % Construct full path for cross-platform compatibility.
        fileName = fullfile(filePath, fileName);
    end

    % Extract base filename for naming outputs.
    [outputPath, baseName, ~] = fileparts(fileName);

    % Open the .wav file.
    [y, fs] = audioread(fileName);
    length_ms = floor(length(y) / fs * 1000);

    % Use file length to determine sequence of gates to create.
    gates = gateSize:gateSize:length_ms;

    % Iterate over each gate, outputting the resultant stimulus.
    for g = gates
        tempY = clipgate(y, fs, g);
        tempName = [fullfile(outputPath, baseName), num2str(g), '.wav'];
        audiowrite(tempName, tempY, fs);
    end

end
```

Combined, the above `.m` files allow one to (nearly) instantly generate a series of gated stimuli from any `.wav` file containing the stimulus of interest. However, gating experiments often involve dozens, if not hundreds, of stimuli, which may be presented under different conditions. Listing 4–12 demonstrates iteration over a list of file names.

Listing 4–12. Function to produce gated stimuli from multiple sound files

```
function gatemultiple()
% GATEMULTIPLE Generate gated stimuli from multiple files.

    % Select multiple files in GUI chooser.
    [files, pathName] = uigetfile('*.wav', 'Select files...', ...
        'MultiSelect', 'on');
```

```
    % Iterate over each file. Note the use of cell-array indexing.
    for f = 1:length(files)
        fileName = fullfile(pathName, files{f});
        allgates('fileName', fileName);
    end

end
```

We now turn our attention to the type of experiment conducted by Lindfield, Wingfield, and Goodglass (1999), in which gated words are presented under three experimental conditions: gated word onset only, word onset plus duration, and word onset plus prosody. The first condition uses stimuli as generated above. The second uses RMS-normalized white noise in place of the remainder of the word. That is, for a 100-ms gate of a 700-ms word, 100 ms of the word are presented, followed directly by 600 ms of white noise. The third condition uses a 325-Hz low-pass filter for the remainder of the word, which has been shown to obscure phonetic information while preserving relevant prosodic properties such as stress and syllable count (Lindfield et al., 1999). A variety of filter designs are reasonable for this purpose; here, we use the `designfilt()` function to allow MATLAB to automatically specify an appropriate design based on the passband and roll-off characteristics desired. This task uses an updated version of the `allgates()` function which accepts an optional parameter for gating type. Note the offloading of complexity to modular back-end functions; the main file-selection and looping program remains simple. The `strcmpi()` function is used to compare condition codes without regard to case. See Listing 4–13.

Listing 4–13. Functions to produce gated stimuli in different experimental conditions

```
function gatecondition(cond)
% GATECONDITION Generate gated stimuli under a specified condition.

    % Handle default condition.
    if nargin < 1
        cond = 'onset';
    end
```

```
    % Select multiple files in GUI chooser.
    [files, pathName] = uigetfile('*.wav', 'Select files...', ...
        'MultiSelect', 'on');
    if ~iscell(files)
        files = {files};
    end

    % Iterate over each file. Note the use of cell-array indexing and the
    % passing of the cond argument to the allgates() function call.
    for f = 1:length(files)
        fileName = fullfile(pathName, files{f});
        allgates2('fileName', fileName, 'condition', cond);
    end

end

function allgates2(varargin)
% ALLGATES2 Generate a set of gated stimuli from a .wav file.

    % Process input arguments.
    p = inputParser();
    p.addParameter('fileName', '');
    p.addParameter('gateSize', 50);
    p.addParameter('condition', 'onset');
    p.parse(varargin{:});
    fileName = p.Results.fileName;
    gateSize = p.Results.gateSize;
    cond = p.Results.condition;

    % If no filename is provided, prompt user for one.
    if isempty(fileName)
        [fileName, filePath] = uigetfile('*.wav', 'Open stimulus file...');

        % Check that a file was selected.
        if isempty(fileName)
            return
        end

        % Construct full path for cross-platform compatibility.
        fileName = fullfile(filePath, fileName);
    end
```

```
% Extract base filename for naming outputs.
[outputPath, baseName, ~] = fileparts(fileName);

% Open the .wav file.
[y, fs] = audioread(fileName);
length_ms = floor(length(y) / fs * 1000);

% Use file length to determine sequence of gates to create.
gates = gateSize:gateSize:length_ms;

% Construct a new filter based on fs, if in the prosody condition.
if strcmpi(cond, 'prosody')
    lpFilt = designfilt('lowpassiir', ...
        'FilterOrder', 8, ...
        'PassbandFrequency', 325, ...
        'SampleRate', fs, ...
        'PassbandRipple', 0.1);
end

% Iterate over each gate, outputting the resultant stimulus. Depending
% on the condition, we alter the way in which the stimulus is created.
for g = gates
    gate_samples = round(g * fs / 1000);

    % Onset plus duration condition.
    if strcmpi(cond, 'duration')
        tempY = y;
        noise = rand(length(y) - gate_samples + 1, 1) * 2 - 1;
        noise = noise .* rms(tempY) ./ rms(noise);
        tempY(gate_samples:end) = noise;

    % Onset plus prosody condition.
    elseif strcmpi(cond, 'prosody')
        tempY = y;
        % Filter with 325-Hz lowpass filter from above code.
        filteredY = filter(lpFilt, y(gate_samples:end));
        % Replace final portion of y with filtered offset.
        tempY(gate_samples:end) = filteredY;
```

```
        % Default, or "onset", condition.
        else
            tempY = clipgate(y, fs, g);
        end

        % Write file including condition name.
        tempName = [fullfile(outputPath, baseName), '-', ...
        num2str(g), ' (', cond, ').wav'];
        audiowrite(tempName, tempY, fs);
    end

end
```

Exercises

1. By modifying only one of the above `.m` files, create a workflow to perform backward gating. That is, your new program should first output the *last* 50 ms of a word, followed by the last 100, and so forth, all the way until the gate closest to the onset is reached.
2. Modify the above programs to keep track of the length of each word in milliseconds, and then output that length into an Excel file.
3. Automate the assignment of words to experimental conditions by writing a script or function which imports an Excel file containing one column of conditions and another column of words. This script will then iterate over each word and select the appropriate processing algorithm to generate the gated stimuli.

Silent-Center Syllables

The silent-center syllable paradigm (Strange, Jenkins, & Johnson, 1983) has long supported the notion that syllable onsets and offsets contain useful information for vowel identification (Jenkins & Strange, 1999). Recent work has expanded this paradigm to bilingual research, examining how the amount of information varies with language experience (Rogers & Lopez, 2008). Silent-center stimuli can be used for word retrieval exercises and cueing techniques, as well as for stimulation; in this way, they provide an alternative to initial-phoneme exercises by also including some rhyme/offset information.

Listing 4–14 demonstrates the creation of silent-center stimuli under a variety of conditions (e.g., Strange et al., 1983), using a master spreadsheet to indicate measured vowel onsets and offsets in milliseconds. We assume that all files have a sampling frequency of 44100 Hz, and are located in the subfolder "Sounds." Note also that we handle conditions in a certain order: we first construct the onset-only and offset-only waveforms, and then use these to build fixed-duration silent-center syllables.

Listing 4–14. Producing silent-center syllables under various conditions

```
% Prompt user for stimulus file.
[fileName, filePath] = uigetfile('*.xlsx', 'Select Stimulus File');
fullFileName = fullfile(filePath,fileName);
[num,txt,raw] = xlsread(fullFileName);

% Assume sampling rate for all files is 44100;
fs = 44100;

% Convert ms to samples;
num = round(num*fs/1000);

% Extract vowel start and stop positions.
vowelStart = num(:,1);
vowelStop = num(:,2);

% Compute duration of vowel.
duration = vowelStop - vowelStart;

% Determine min and max durations for length matching.
minDuration = min(duration);
maxDuration = max(duration);

% Determine number of wave files to analyze.
[numFiles, numColumns] = size(num);

% Iterate.
for i = 1:numFiles

    % Load wave file and get base filename for outputs.
    wavName = fullfile(filePath, 'Sounds', txt{i+1,1});
    [PATHSTR, BaseName] = fileparts(wavName);
    y = audioread(wavName);
```

```
% Extract the current file's vowel start and stop points.
tempStart = vowelStart(i);
tempStop = vowelStop(i);

% Condition 1 - No change.
temp = y;
saveName = fullfile(PATHSTR,[BaseName,num2str(1),'.wav']);
audiowrite(saveName, temp, fs)

% Condition 2 - Silent center, original duration;
temp = y;
saveName = fullfile(PATHSTR,[BaseName,num2str(2),'.wav']) ;
temp(tempStart:tempStop) = 0;
audiowrite(saveName, temp, fs)

% Condition 3 - Center only, original duration;
temp = y;
saveName = fullfile(PATHSTR,[BaseName,num2str(3),'.wav']) ;
temp(1:tempStart) = 0;
temp(tempStop:end) = 0;
audiowrite(saveName, temp, fs)

% Condition 4 - Center only, fixed duration;
temp = y;
saveName = fullfile(PATHSTR,[BaseName,num2str(4),'.wav']);
temp(1:tempStart) = 0;
fixedStop = tempStart + minDuration;
temp(fixedStop:end) = 0;
audiowrite(saveName, temp, fs)

% Condition 7 - Onset only;
tempInitial = y;
saveName = fullfile(PATHSTR,[BaseName,num2str(7),'.wav']);
tempInitial = tempInitial(1:tempStart);
audiowrite(saveName, tempInitial, fs)

% Condition 8 - Offset only;
tempFinal = y;
saveName = fullfile(PATHSTR,[BaseName,num2str(8),'.wav']);
tempFinal = tempFinal(tempStop:end);
audiowrite(saveName, tempFinal, fs)
```

```
    % Condition 5 - Silent center, short duration;
    temp = [tempInitial;zeros(minDuration,1);tempFinal];
    saveName = fullfile(PATHSTR,[BaseName,num2str(5),'.wav']);
    audiowrite(saveName, temp, fs)

    % Condition 6 - Silent center, long duration;
    temp = [tempInitial;zeros(maxDuration,1);tempFinal];
    saveName = fullfile(PATHSTR,[BaseName,num2str(6),'.wav']);
    audiowrite(saveName, temp, fs)

end
```

Exercises

1. The above program assumes a constant sampling rate. Adjust it so that it can handle files of different sampling rates.
2. Rewrite the program to use a table object instead of a separate numeric and character variables.
3. The process used for naming and saving files is repetitive. Create a separate function that handles this process. Hint: Consider passing the path string, the base filename, a number, and the audio data as arguments to this function.

Stereo and Multichannel Audio

Presentation of audio to one of two stereo channels, or to one of several sound-field channels, is of great use in auditory perception experiments and in hearing screenings. By calibrating a set of headphones and their attached sound card, it is possible to construct custom audiogram equipment in MATLAB.

As discussed in earlier chapters, audio is represented in MATLAB by a $s \times c$ matrix, where s denotes the number of samples and c the number of channels. A monaural audio recording will consist of a single column of numbers, whereas a stereo audio recording will have two concurrent columns. A monaural audio matrix can easily be converted into stereo through the use of the `repmat()` function as in Listing 4–15. Column 1 represents the left channel, whereas column 2 represents the right. Note that a separate function is usually not needed for most applications but is provided as a pedagogical example.

Listing 4–15. Conversion from mono to stereo

```
function y = mono2stereo(y)
% MONO2STEREO Convert a mono file to stereo.

    % Check size of y, since it may already be stereo or multichannel.
    [rows, cols] = size(y);
    if cols >= 2 && rows > 1 % Already stereo, so do nothing;
        return
    end

    % Ensure y is a column vector.
    y = y(:);

    % Duplicate mono channel to left and right.
    y = repmat(y, 1, 2);

end
```

Audiological testing requires presentation of stimuli to each ear individually, and at varying amplitudes. This can be done by zeroing out the opposite column of the audio matrix: to present to the right ear only, we zero out the left column, and vice versa. The example in Listing 4–16 generates a 1000-Hz sine wave at half of the current volume setting and plays it to the left ear first, then to the right. Note the use of the `fliplr()` function to switch channels.

Listing 4–16. Playing to the left and right ear in succession

```
% Generate a 1000-Hz sine tone (monaural).
fs = 44100;
time = (1:fs) / fs;
y = 0.5 * sin(2*pi*1000*time);

% Duplicate to stereo.
y = mono2stereo(y);
```

```
% Play to left ear.
input('Press ENTER to play to left ear: ');
yLeft = y;
yLeft(:, 2) = 0;
sound(yLeft, fs)

% Play to right ear
input('Press ENTER to play to right ear: ');
yRight = fliplr(yLeft);
sound(yRight, fs)
```

It is also possible to play a sound sample to both ears simultaneously, but with different amplitudes. To do this, we simply multiply each channel by its own scaling factor (<1). This can be done from a monaural input signal with matrix multiplication as in Listing 4–17, or from a stereo signal as in Listing 4–18.

Listing 4–17. Matrix multiplication for different amplitudes

```
% Generate a 1000-Hz sine tone (monaural).
fs = 44100;
time = (1:fs) / fs;
y = sin(2*pi*1000*time);

% Define channel amplitudes as a 1x2 matrix.
amps = [0.5, 0.1];

% Transpose so we have a Sx1 matrix (audio) to be
% multiplied by a 1x2 matrix (amplitudes).
y = y';

% Matrix multiplication
% Sx1 times 1x2 gives an Sx2 matrix.
y = y * amps;
```

Listing 4–18. Applying different amplitudes to a stereo matrix

```
% Generate a 1000-Hz sine tone (monaural).
fs = 44100;
time = (1:fs) / fs;
y = 0.5 * sin(2*pi*1000*time);

% Duplicate to stereo.
y = mono2stereo(y);

% Define channel amplitudes.
amps = [0.5, 0.1];

% Replicate amplitudes for length of signal.
amps = repmat(amps, length(y), 1);

% Apply elementwise multiplication.
y = amps .* y;
```

With appropriate external modules or Toolboxes, MATLAB can also play multichannel audio. This is particularly useful in constructing sound-fields in three-dimensional space. When working with multichannel audio, each column of the audio matrix represents a separate channel, just as in stereo audio. However, the traditional assignment of left versus right no longer applies; instead, the physical meaning of each channel is left to the clinician or investigator.

One common setup involves the placement of an array of speakers at different azimuth angles from the listener or participant. Another involves the creation of a three-dimensional speaker cube, as in surround-sound applications. Finally, the most complex systems will involve large panels of speakers in an anechoic chamber, which play phase-shifted variants of a signal such that the listener perceives the sound source to be a point in three-dimensional space.

The example presented in Listing 4–19 assumes that we have a left-front, right-front, left-back, and right-back channel (four-channel setup), and that the channels are in that order. We synthesize a 440-Hz sine tone and play it from each channel in turn, effecting a "zig-zag" sound source. This example uses the `pa_wavplay()` function (Frear, 2004) to access multichannel hardware. While the setup of particular hardware systems is beyond the scope of this text, most if not all multichannel sound cards ship with instructions on how to access this feature.

Listing 4–19. Multichannel audio presentation

```
% Generate a monaural 440-Hz tone.
fs = 44100;
time = (1:fs)' / fs;
tone = sin(2*pi*440*time);

% Set up a 4-channel template for each stimulus. This assumes
% we have 4 channels, as stated in the text.
yBase = zeros(fs, 4);
y1 = yBase;
y2 = yBase;
y3 = yBase;
y4 = yBase;

% Set up each stimulus wave independently. We do this by copying
% the base tone to the appropriate channel. For larger numbers
% of channels, we would automate this with a FOR loop.
y1(:, 1) = tone;
y2(:, 2) = tone;
y3(:, 3) = tone;
y4(:, 4) = tone;

% Play each wave in turn.
input('Press ENTER for front-left sound: ');
pa_wavplay(y1, fs);
input('Press ENTER for front-right sound: ');
pa_wavplay(y2, fs);
input('Press ENTER for back-left sound: ');
pa_wavplay(y3, fs);
input('Press ENTER for back-right sound: ');
pa_wavplay(y4, fs);
```

Exercises

1. If we wanted to test perception of speech sounds from the front versus the back, how might we implement this using only a stereo-capable sound card?
2. Create a pair of functions `presentToLeft()` and `presentToRight()` that accept a column vector and present it to the indicated channel.

3. Generalize the above functions to a `presentToChannel()` function, which accepts a column vector of sound data the specified channel, and the total number of channels.
4. Suppose we have a panning vector whose values range from 0 (left) to 1 (right). Assume this vector is of the same length as a desired stimulus. Create a function that accepts a monaural column vector and the panning vector mentioned above, and apply the panning such that (a) the total amplitude of both channels equals the amplitude of the original signal, and (b) the proportion of the signal in the right channel corresponds to the panning vector.

Data Collection and Analysis

Speech, language, and hearing assessments involve the quantification of parameters derived from speech, language, and hearing samples. Sampling and/or assessment can be at the level of the phone, phoneme, syllable, morpheme, word, foot, meter, utterance, or even paragraph. Test formats can be open and semistructured, as may occur during bedside evaluation or in play settings, or they may include published tests such as the Goldman-Fristoe Test of Articulation 2 (Goldman & Fristoe, 2000; Goldman, Fristoe, & Woodcock, 1971), the Peabody Picture Vocabulary Test, Fourth Edition (Dunn & Dunn, 2007), or the Western Aphasia Battery-Revised (Kertesz, 2006), to name a few. For improved automaticity, however, it may well be advisable to design test stimuli better suited to extraction of parameters. As an example, vowel durations and properties are more easily computed when vowels are contrasted mainly with voiceless stops; when glides and approximants are included in reading samples, automated vowel extraction can prove intractable.

Recording Sounds

Assuming a clean audio chain including a quality microphone and/or headset, optional pre-amplifier, and sound card, a direct acoustic representation of a patient's speech sample can be recorded using an `audiorecorder` object as outlined in the following listing. For convenience, sample code is reproduced in Listing 4–20 to capture a speech sample with standard 44100 Hz sampling rate, 16-bit precision, and monaural input. This code will create (among others) two variables in the MATLAB Workspace: `y` (the audio data) and `fs` (indicating sampling rate). Note that this will overwrite any variables with the same name.

Listing 4–20. Recording a sound in MATLAB

```
% Set recording parameters for typical CD audio.
fs = 44100;
nbits = 16;

% Create audiorecorder object.
ar = audiorecorder(fs, nbits, 1);

% Prompt for start and stop of recording.
input('Press ENTER to begin recording: ')
record(ar)
input('Press ENTER to stop recording: ')
stop(ar)

% Extract speech signal.
y = getaudiodata(ar);
```

This recording can be replayed by entering `play(ar)` in the Command Window. Note that unlike the `sound()` function, which requires specification of sampling rate, `play()` automatically determines the sampling rate of the speech sample by querying the corresponding property of the `audiorecorder` object. The same effect can be achieved by entering the command `sound(y, fs)`.

Exercises

1. Encapsulate the above features into a function that accepts a sampling frequency as an input argument and returns the signal.
2. Using the `audiowrite()` function, create a function to record a sound sample and then to save it to a file. Allow the user to select this file with the `uiputfile()` function.

Plotting Sound Wave Forms

It is often useful to plot the waveform of a speech sound, both for data quality purposes and for closer inspection of patterns of interest (Figure 4–3). Although `plot()` can serve this purpose, the default plotting function will use the index (sample number) as the horizontal coordinate. In viewing speech

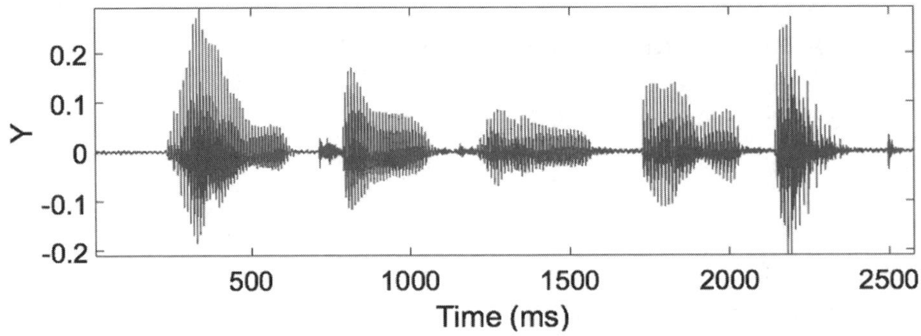

Figure 4–3. Waveform plot.

data, it is preferable to see time rather than index on the horizontal axis, mainly for the purpose of measuring durations of speech segments. Listing 4–21 illustrates a more "complete" plotting solution. It assumes that we have a variable `y` containing the speech data, and `fs` specifying the sampling rate.

Listing 4–21. Plotting an existing waveform

```
% Create time vector in milliseconds.
time = (1:length(y)) / fs * 1000;

% Plot the waveform with respect to time.
plot(time, y);
xlabel('Time (ms)')
ylabel('Y')
```

Exercise

1. Create a function that accepts a column vector and sample rate, and then performs the above plotting commands.

Plotting Sound Frequencies: Spectra and Spectrograms

The amplitude spectrum of a speech signal is used to determine the amplitudes of its component frequencies (Figure 4–4). Computation of spectra constitutes a preliminary step for a wide variety of speech analyses employed in clinical and research practice.

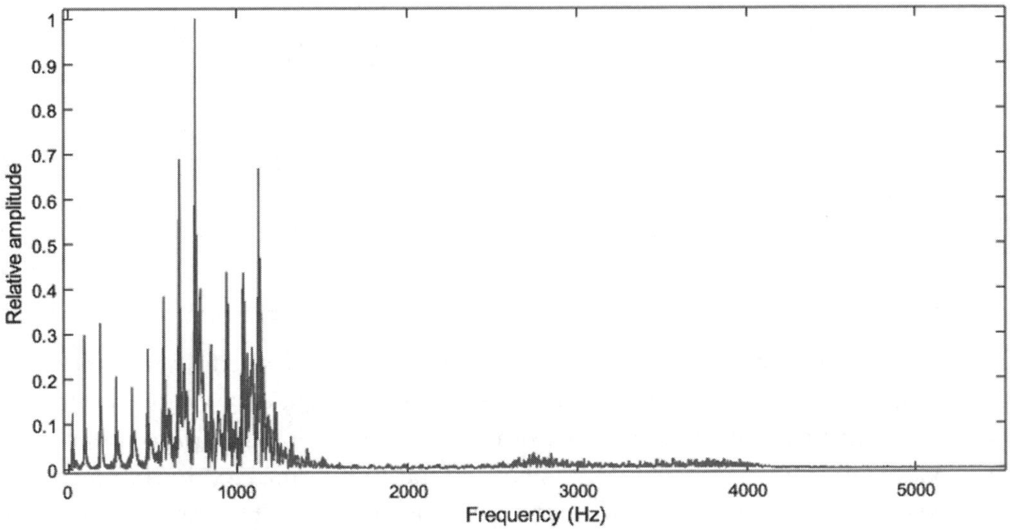

Figure 4–4. Amplitude spectrum (zoomed in to 0–5000 Hz).

In MATLAB, a simple way to obtain an amplitude spectrum is the `fft()` function. FFT stands for "fast Fourier transform" and is a computationally efficient way to estimate the magnitude of the signal's components. Listing 4–22 demonstrates the application of this technique to speech data.

Listing 4–22. Computing the FFT and plotting the amplitude spectrum of a signal

```
% Get length of signal.
L = length(y);

% Determine FFT length.
NFFT = 2^nextpow2(L);

% Compute FFT and normalize.
Y = fft(y, NFFT) / L;

% Determine frequencies that are examined.
freqs = fs/2 * linspace(0, 1, NFFT/2 + 1);

% Get absolute magnitude of the complex transform.
amps = 2*abs(Y(1:NFFT/2+1));
```

```
% Compute relative amplitudes (set max component to 1).
amps = amps ./ max(amps);

% Plot amplitude spectrum.
plot(freqs, amps)
xlabel('Frequency (Hz)')
ylabel('Relative amplitude')
```

By its very nature, speech varies over time and so does its acoustic footprint. As such, it would not be reasonable to expect a single spectrum to capture information that is representative. If we consider a spectrum as a "snapshot" in time, a spectrogram is somewhat like a "movie," in that it traces the evolution of the spectrum over time (Figure 4–5). The `spectrogram()` function allows one to plot a spectrogram of a speech signal, as illustrated

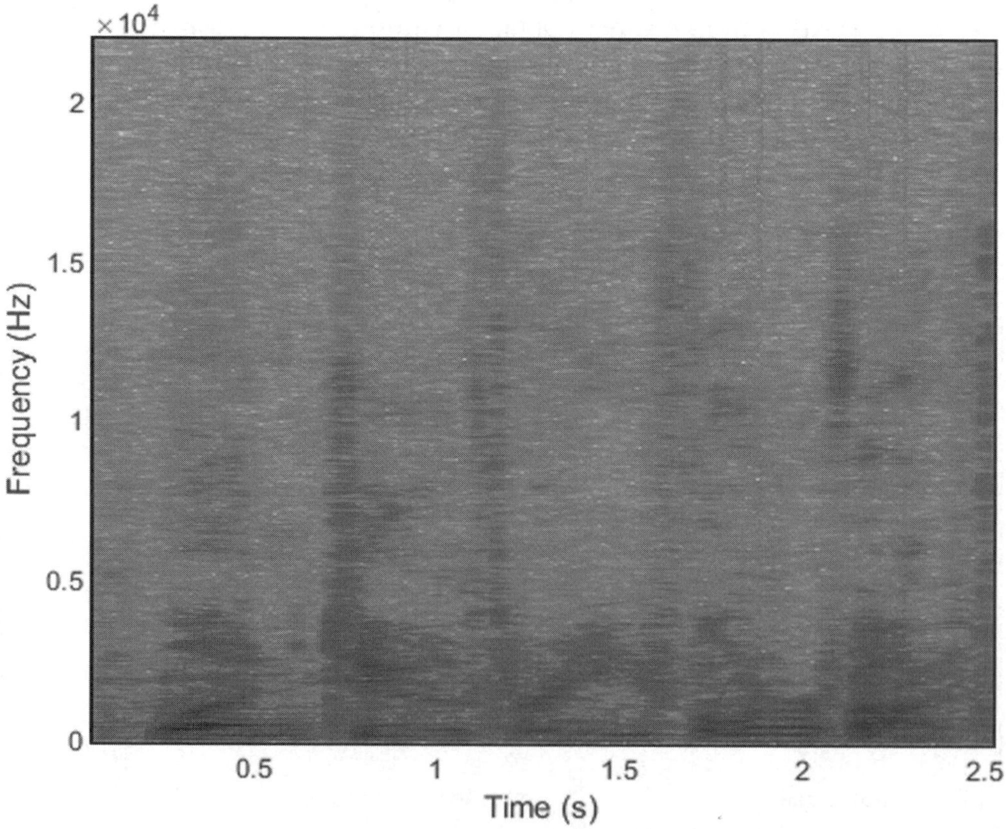

Figure 4–5. Example spectrogram output from the `spectrogram()` function.

below, by taking successive windowed spectra. Because of its complexity, additional parameters must be specified, such as the window length and the amount of overlap. See Listing 4–23.

Listing 4–23. Generation of a spectrogram

```
% Compute window size of 100 ms.
win = round(fs * 0.1);

% Use overlap of 90 ms.
overlap = round(fs * 0.09);

% Plot a spectrogram with time on the x-axis
% and frequency on the y-axis.
spectrogram(y, win, overlap, 1024, fs, 'yaxis');
```

The listing in Appendix D, depicted in Figure 4–6, demonstrates the programmatic specification of a simple spectral analysis GUI, which can be used to great effect in interactive speech-science demonstrations. Such GUIs can also be designed using the GUIDE utility included in MATLAB.

Detecting and Analyzing Formants

Formants are regions of higher energy in a spectrum, and are associated with resonant frequencies of the vocal tract. Fant (1960) defines formants as "the spectral peaks of the sound spectrum." As with pitch, formants also vary across time, and it is of interest to clinicians and speech scientists alike to estimate this variation by tracking the main formant frequencies of speech. In particular, the first two formants are sufficient for most listeners to identify a vowel (e.g., Stevens, 2000), and in this way are considered to carry the largest portion of that vowel's identity. Furthermore, formant transitions in consonantal contexts assist in identification of the consonant in terms of a common locus frequency (Kent & Read, 1992).

Clinical uses of formant tracking include training for articulation of vowels, provision of visual feedback in articulation exercises, and assessing deterioration of the patient's vowel space due to age or disease. Patients can be shown acoustic targets by way of formant plots and encouraged to reach them, assisting in clearer speech.

Formant tracking generally proceeds by way of identifying the changing location of spectral peaks in a spectrogram. A useful algorithm for extracting

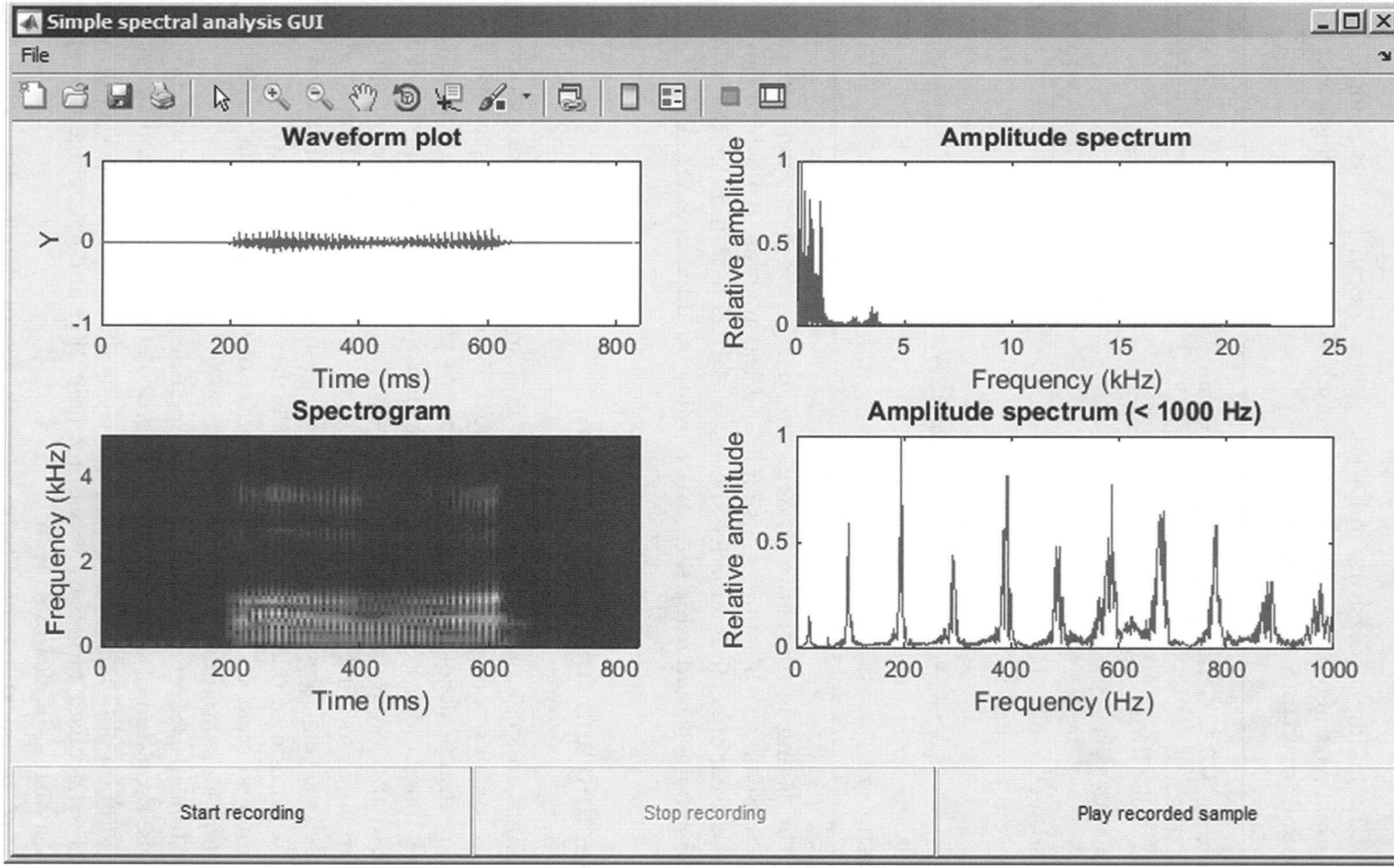

Figure 4–6. Example session of the spectral analysis GUI.

formant peaks is known as linear predictive coding (LPC) (O'Shaughnessy, 1988). In some ways, LPC analysis is an inverse of the source-filter model, in that it begins with a signal already "filtered" by the vocal tract and attempts to determine the coefficients of a second filter that cancels the signal (Ladefoged, 1996). The peaks in the LPC spectrum correspond closely to formants of the vocal tract, with the caveat that the additional filtering performed by lip radiation is also included.

LPC analysis can be done with the `lpc()` function included in the Signal Processing Toolbox. Listing 4–24 demonstrates the extraction of the first two formants, which warrants the use of a sixth-order model—in general, the order is specified as $2n + 2$, where n is the number of formants one wishes to extract (Snell & Milinazzo, 1993). Assume we have a signal stored in the variable `y`, and the sampling frequency stored in `fs`. Further assume that we have identified a central or stable period of a vowel, whose onset and offset times in milliseconds are stored in `onset_ms` and `offset_ms`.

Listing 4–24. Detection of formant frequencies

```
% Convert milliseconds to samples.
onset = round(onset / 1000 * fs);
offset = round(offset / 1000 * fs);

% Extract central portion of the vowel.
ySegment = y(onset:offset);

% Apply a window to avoid spectral splatter.
w = hamming(length(ySegment));
ySegment = w .* ySegment;

% Perform LPC modeling.
nFormants = 2;
lpcCoeffs = lpc(ySegment, nFormants * 2 + 2);

% Find the roots of the LPC polynomial, ignoring complex conjugates.
lpcRoots = roots(lpcCoeffs);
lpcRoots = lpcRoots(imag(lpcRoots) >= 0);

% Compute angle from origin and convert to frequency.
angles = atan2(imag(lpcRoots), real(lpcRoots));
freqs = angles .* fs / (2*pi);
```

To determine the acoustic distance from one vowel to the next, within a speaker, a common approach is to compare F1 and F2 values in a two-dimensional Euclidean space. This means that we plot F1 on one axis, F2 on another, and compute the distance between two (F1, F2) coordinate pairs. Across speakers, this approach is also useful albeit more limited owing to regions of overlap in this F1–F2 space.

To account for the logarithmic nature of pitch perception, we can adjust the distance computation by converting the linear units of Hz into logarithmic units of cents (1/100 of a semitone). These units correspond more closely with the nature of human speech perception. In Listing 4–25, the function takes two vectors of formants as input and computes the distance between them in terms of cents.

Listing 4–25. Function to compute formant distances

```
function d = formantdistance(v1Formants, v2Formants)

    % Ensure both vectors are column vectors.
    v1Formants = v1Formants(:);
    v2Formants = v2Formants(:);

    % Abort if the sizes don't match.
    if length(v1Formants) ~= length(v2Formants)
       error('Unequal number of formants (%d vs %d)', ...
          length(v1Formants), length(v2Formants));
    end

    % Compute component distances in cents. Note the use of ./ for
    % elementwise, not matrix, division.
    dCents = 1200*log2(v2Formants ./ v1Formants);

    % Compute Euclidean distance.
    % Note that this assumes each formant dimension
    % is weighted equally.
    d = sqrt(sum(dCents.^2));

end
```

Measures of Voice Quality

Voice quality is a parameter that is influenced by a person's vocal tract anatomy, articulatory configuration, and motor execution. Because of this complexity, capturing voice quality has eluded clinicians and researchers alike. Moreover, reliance on subjective assessments of voice quality has led to the use of a variety of labels compounding the lack of reliability inherent in subjective assessment. Titze (1994) has identified at least 25 different terms denoting voice quality which may have overlapping or conflicting meanings. Furthermore, reliability even in the same rater has been found lacking (Stellars et al., 2009).

Objective measures of voice quality derive from acoustic analysis, which often has been the response province of closed-source, turn-key software. Such tools, convenient as they may be, afford researchers and clinicians little control over how the analysis is conducted. This section details more "open" methods in MATLAB for computing voice quality measures, or components thereof, from patients' speech samples.

A commonly used measure of voice quality is the SNR, also known as the harmonics-to-noise ratio or speech-to-noise ratio. In disordered voices, this ratio is lower, indicating greater levels of noise (Colton & Casper, 2011). One must be careful to contrast this voice-internal SNR from the SNR arising from a poorly configured recording setup; if noise arises from the equipment itself, precise measurement of the patient's voice characteristics becomes difficult if not impossible. Furthermore, since the "noise" against which we are comparing the speech portion of the signal is part of the speech itself, several operational definitions of SNR exist. This section will use the NIST (Fillinger, 2008) definition of speech-to-noise ratio.

The SNR can be computed with functions available in the Signal Processing Toolbox (MathWorks, 2015), as well as with several freely available toolboxes and functions. This process involves comparing the overall spectral content of the signal in regions containing speech as compared to those which do not (e.g., Karam, Khazaal, Aglan, & Cole, 2014). Speech detection can be automatized through the VOICEBOX set of routines (Brookes, 2013), in particular, the Sohn voice activity detector (`vadsohn.m`). Listing 4–26 assumes that the VOICEBOX routines have been downloaded to the "VOICEBOX" folder in the user's MATLAB working directory, and uses the formula $SNR_{dB}=20 \times \log_{10}(RMS_{YS}/RMS_{YN})$, where YS denotes the section of the recording with identified speech and YN the section with nonspeech or noise (cf. Quantieri, 2001).

Listing 4–26. Computing SNR

```
% Add VOICEBOX files to path.
addpath('VOICEBOX');

% Use VOICEBOX to detect voice activity.
% Note: This uses default settings, but can be customized
% to a particular clinical or research application.
% The output argument vs contains a 1 for each sample
% in a speech region, and a 0 for each sample in a
% non-speech or noise region.
vs = vadsohn(y, fs);

% Plot original wave and voice activity.
% Useful for manual verification of speech detection.
time = (1:length(y)) / fs;
plot(time, y)
axis tight
ylim([-1.1, 1.1])
hold on
plot(time, vs)

% Determine RMS amplitude for speech and non-speech regions.
% These computations use logical indexing based on the detected regions
% in vs.
rmsSpeech = rms(y(vs == 1));
rmsNonSpeech = rms(y(vs == 0));

% Compute SNR in dB.
snrdb = 20*log10(rmsSpeech / rmsNonSpeech);
```

Prosody

Over the past several decades, limited theoretical guidance has emerged in regard to quantifying prosody. The Mixdorff-Fujisaki model (Fujisaki & Hirose, 1984; Mixdorff, 2000), for example, has been used to describe f0 contours extracted from speech signals. In the domain of transcription, the tones and break indices (ToBI; Pierrehumbert, 1980; Silverman et al., 1992) are a simplified system for indicating (i.e., tagging) tonal and boundary aspects of a speech utterance.

Several recent studies have attempted to quantify multiple dimensions at once. For example, Patel and Campellone (2009) examined pitch, duration, and intensity as separate response variables in terms of contrastive stress in persons with dysarthria. Unfortunately, while prosody is most likely more than the simple sum of intensity, pitch, and duration (pauses), prosodic theories often treat these dimensions separately without putting them back together, as it were.

Furthermore, clinical assessment of prosody is currently impressionistic at best, as the psychophysical quantification of prosody is still lacking. As a result, the contribution of these cues to perception when combined is not known, and nor are the levels/thresholds for saliency, perceptual prominence, or prosodic disorders. Today, most theories focus on intonation (pitch) and define hierarchical levels of prosody without specifying thresholds. That said, computerized analysis of speech could facilitate the development of such guidelines, which would prove instrumental for assessment and treatment of both prosody perception and production.

In this and the following sections, we discuss applying MATLAB programming techniques to generate amplitude envelopes, detect speech (voiced and unvoiced) versus silence, perform pitch tracking, and to compute speech and articulation rate. We also offer guidelines for stimulus selection to increase automaticity and accuracy of the analyses.

Intensity Envelopes

When viewing a waveform of speech, it is easy to see that the amplitude of the signal often varies substantially. Some portions of the speech signal may be much louder than others, and yet others (e.g., pauses and stop gaps) may be so silent that they do not rise above the noise floor. To a first approximation, the envelope is essentially the outline of a signal's waveform. In English, changes in the speech amplitude envelope often occur when a syllable is stressed. The variability of the amplitude envelope is a graphical measure of a patient's prosody—an envelope that is too flat could indicate mono-loudness, a symptom of underlying prosodic deficiencies.

The `rms()` function discussed earlier allows amplitude computation across the entire signal, but to visualize the envelope of changing amplitude over time, a more sophisticated approach is needed. Unfortunately, there is no universally agreed standard for computing envelopes; in fact, the technique applied often depends on constraints such as bandwidth, time cost, and processing power (e.g., for real-time applications).

This approach uses the Hilbert transform (1953), which can be used to determine the instantaneous amplitude for a given point in the signal. In MATLAB, when operating on monaural audio sequences, the `hilbert()` function returns a complex-valued vector (see Appendix B for review of complex numbers), termed the *analytic signal*, whose real part is the original signal and whose imaginary part is the actual Hilbert transform. Although the mathematics of this complex-valued transform is beyond the scope of the text, it is well established that taking the magnitude of the analytic signal yields an amplitude envelope. The code in Listing 4–27 illustrates recording a patient's speech sample, taking the Hilbert transform, computing the magnitude of the analytic signal, and plotting the amplitude envelope.

Listing 4–27. Hilbert envelope

```
% Use standard CD-audio settings.
fs = 44100;
nbits = 16;

% Create audiorecorder object.
ar = audiorecorder(fs, nbits, 1);

% Record the sample.
input('Press ENTER to begin recording: ')
record(ar)
input('Press ENTER to stop recording: ')
stop(ar)

% Extract the speech data from the audiorecorder object.
y = getaudiodata(ar);

% Determine time in seconds for each sample point.
time = (1:length(y)) / fs;

% Compute the Hilbert transform.
yh = hilbert(y);

% Compute the magnitude of the complex vector.
% This gives the amplitude envelope.
env = sqrt(real(yh).^2 + imag(yh).^2);
```

```
% Plot the envelope with respect to time.
plot(time, env)
xlabel('Time (s)')
ylabel('Amplitude')
```

In Figure 4–7 are plotted a simple speech signal (a sequence of numbers read aloud) and its corresponding Hilbert envelope, as computed with the above code. It can be seen that the Hilbert envelope corresponds broadly with the waveform's outline, as desired. Such a result can be further used in MATLAB for things like speech versus nonspeech detection, measurement of pause duration, and so on.

A drawback of this method is that, depending on the sampling rate used, its resolution may be too high and give too much prominence to almost instantaneous acoustic change (i.e., we are often interested in a broader picture of the changing amplitude over time, rather than on the numerous oscillations as seen above). One solution is to apply a smoothing algorithm to the data stored in `env`, as in Listing 4–28 (Figure 4–8). This uses the concept of a moving-average filter implemented through convolution, as discussed in **Chapter 2**. Here we use a window with an odd number of samples so that

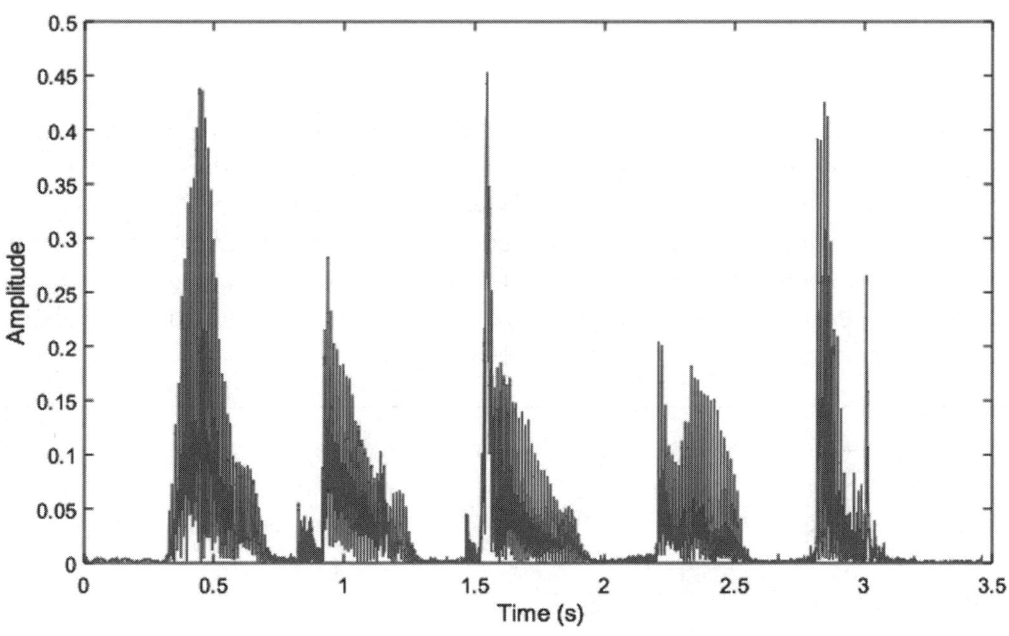

Figure 4–7. Plot of a Hilbert transformed signal.

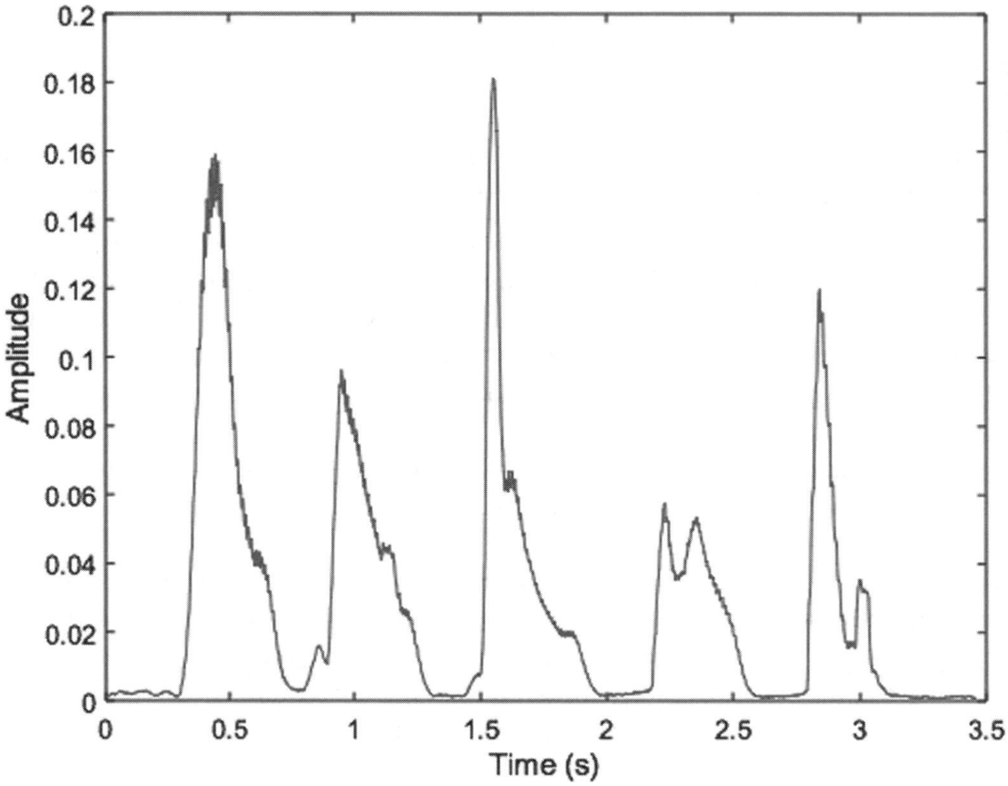

Figure 4–8. A plot of a smoothed amplitude envelope.

the computed average can be stored in the exact center. The window size is informed by the fact that, on the order of 50 ms or so, the human vocal tract can be considered approximately stationary (Smith, 2002). The `'same'` parameter is supplied to the `conv` function to inform MATLAB that we want a sequence of the same length as the original signal. Often, it is the relative changes in amplitude over time that are of importance rather than the absolute numerical values attained by the envelope.

Listing 4–28. Applying a smoothing algorithm

```
% Estimate desired window radius based on total size of 50 ms
% at the given sampling frequency.
windowRad = ceil((0.05 * fs) / 2);
windowSize = 2*windowRad + 1;
```

```
% Set up moving-average window. Assume y is a column vector.
win = ones(windowSize, 1) / windowSize;

% Convolve the window with our envelope signal. Use the 'same' option
% to keep the envelope at the same number of samples.
envSmoothed = conv(env, win, 'same');
plot(time, envSmoothed)
xlabel('Time (s)')
ylabel('Amplitude')
```

Exercises

1. What would occur if we applied a moving-window average with a very large window size? How might this affect our visualization of amplitude peaks?
2. If we compute the RMS of the entire signal, we do not acquire the amplitude envelope, but we do gain some information. What does this information tell us about the speaker, assuming we use consistent microphone settings from one patient to the next?
3. Suppose we wish to quantify a patient's amplitude variability. Using the `std()` function to compute standard deviation, write a function that accepts a signal `y` and sampling rate `fs`, and returns a measure of variability in the patient's amplitude envelope. Interpret this measure.

Detection of Speech Versus Silence: Pauses

Usage of the `vadsohn()` function (Brookes, 2003) allows for easy detection of speech versus silence in a speech signal, as might occur in a conversational sample or in a passage reading exercise. Most of the silence in speech can be attributed to pauses, but some silence may occur between recording onset and speech onset, or between speech offset and recording offset. The silence attributed to pauses is meaningful and should be preserved, but the silence simply due to microphone timing on the part of the clinician or investigator is likely of no interest, and can be discarded.

Pauses normally occur at grammatically appropriate places in the speech signal, and help listeners parse the constituents of an utterance in the manner that is intended by the speaker. Pauses also occur for a variety of other reasons, such as uncertainty, lack of ideation, formulation and/or word retrieval difficulty, initiation of repair, as well as pausing for pragmatic effect.

Therefore, detection of pauses in speech can be very useful in documenting some of the aforementioned processes in speech. In addition, if pauses are added together, the summed pause time can be subtracted from total spoken time so that, in turn, articulation rate can be derived. Specifically, the total articulation time is used as the denominator, rather than total signal length. Knowing the number of syllables of a passage is helpful in this regard; however, we will later explore how to estimate this number, especially for CV sequences as in diadochokinetic tasks.

Listing 4–29 assumes that the VOICEBOX toolbox (Brookes, 2003) has been installed and is located in the "VOICEBOX" folder. Source code for VOICEBOX can be found at http://www.ee.ic.ac.uk/hp/staff/dmb/voicebox/voicebox.html. This program assumes the signal is stored in `y` and its sampling rate in `fs`, and returns a vector of ones and zeros, corresponding to speech and silent regions, respectively.

Listing 4–29. Detection of speech versus silence

```
% Add VOICEBOX files to path.
addpath('VOICEBOX');

% Use VOICEBOX to detect voice activity.
% Note: This uses default settings, but can be customized
% to a particular clinical or research application.
% The output argument vs contains a 1 for each sample
% in a speech region, and a 0 for each sample in a
% non-speech or noise region.
vs = vadsohn(y, fs);

% Plot original wave and voice activity.
time = (1:length(y)) / fs;
plot(time, y)
axis tight
ylim([-1.1, 1.1])
hold on
plot(time, vs)
```

Exercises

1. Use the above code to produce a function that accepts a signal `y` and a sampling rate `fs`, then returns the total articulation time in milliseconds.
2. Design a function that returns a copy of a signal `y`, but removes the silences at the beginning and end.
3. Using Listing 4–29 and any combination of the exercises, create a function that computes speech rate and articulation rate for a passage with a known number of syllables. This function should accept a "raw" sound file (with possible silences before speech onset and after speech onset), its sampling rate, and the expected number of syllables for the passage. It should trim leading and trailing pauses to compute speech rate, and then remove medial or interword pauses to compute articulation rate. Use multiple output arguments to return both rates to the user.

Detection of Voicing

After determining which segments of the signal constitute speech via the above code, one might next wish to separate out voiced versus unvoiced sounds. The percentage of unvoiced sounds can be likened to a perturbation factor to the flow of speech, and provides indication of the likelihood of discoordination failure (e.g., a mismatch in intended voicing vs. realized voicing in ostensibly voiceless stops, fricatives, and affricates). Furthermore, this percentage holds promise as an index to rate the "fluency" challenge a reading passage may pose, especially for persons with apraxia of speech (Kent & Rosenbek, 1983) or fluency disorders such as stuttering (Kalveram, 1991).

Voicing detection is also an important component in pitch tracking, as voiceless sounds do not exhibit a fundamental frequency or harmonic structure. Therefore, many pitch tracking algorithms include this detection as a first step. For example, the YAAPT algorithm (Yet Another Algorithm for Pitch Tracking) (Zahorian & Hu, 2008) discussed below automatically returns a sequence of pitches, with values of 0 indicating voiceless and nonzero values indicating estimated pitch in hertz. Listing 4–30 demonstrates the combination of `vadsohn()` for speech versus nonspeech detection, and then `yaapt()` for voiced versus voiceless sounds, and outputs a vector with the following coding: 0 = nonspeech, 1 = voiceless, 2 = voiced. Because both functions return vectors with different sampling rates and timings, a time-track adjustment will be required to reconcile the data streams. As opposed to traditional resampling and interpolation, we use a nearest-neighbor algorithm to keep the values from each data stream discrete.

Listing 4–30. Function to detect voiced versus voiceless sounds

```
function sampleType = detectvoicing(y, fs)
    % Create time vector for synchronization.
    time = (1:length(y)) / fs;

    % Extract pitch using YAAPT.
    % Note that frameLength is in milliseconds.
    [pitch, nf, frameLength] = yaapt(y, fs, 1);
    pitchTime = (1:length(pitch)) * frameLength / 1000;

    % Use VOICEBOX to detect voice activity.
    vs = vadsohn(y, fs);

    % Use YAAPT data to find voicing.
    voiced = double(pitch > 0);

    % Upsample the YAAPT voicing stream using nearest-neighbor.
    voiced2 = interp1(pitchTime, voiced, time, 'nearest');
    voiced2 = voiced2(:);

    % Now the voicing stream and the voice-activity stream have the same
    % number of samples. We compute a combination of the two to yield the
    % desired codes.
    sampleType = (voiced2 .* vs) + vs;

end
```

Pitch Tracking

Aside from amplitude or intensity, prosody also concerns itself with variations in the speaker's voice pitch. These variations are easily perceived as part of the speaker's intonation, and tend to covary with changes in amplitude. However, they can also be estimated in isolation. Furthermore, voice pitch itself is indicative of glottal pulse rate.

The fundamental tool of pitch tracking is autocorrelation. In simple terms, autocorrelation essentially "slides" two copies of a signal past each other, sample by sample, and determines when and where they "line up." The amount of samples by which the signal is shifted relative to itself is termed the *lag*. When the signal lines up with its time-shifted counterpart, the value of the autocorrelation sequence at that lag point is high. If the signal is out of sync at a given lag, the autocorrelation sequence at that point will be close to zero. If the lag causes the signal to be of the opposite sign (i.e., 180 degrees out of phase), the autocorrelation sequence at that point will be negative. Consider the following simplified "speech signal" (a 100-Hz sine tone sampled at 44100 Hz) and its computed autocorrelation sequence (Figures 4–9 and 4–10). Note that technically autocorrelation should be plotted as a function of time, not samples of lag, but the figure is presented to show the raw output from the MATLAB function.

As the sine wave's copy is slid further and further to the right, we can see that the signal will move in and out of phase with itself. At points where the sine waves are in phase, the autocorrelation sequence has a local maximum. This is illustrated in Figure 4–11, with a data cursor indicated for clarity.

From this, it can be determined that the period of repetition is approximately 441 samples, or 10 ms, which implies the fundamental frequency is 100 Hz.

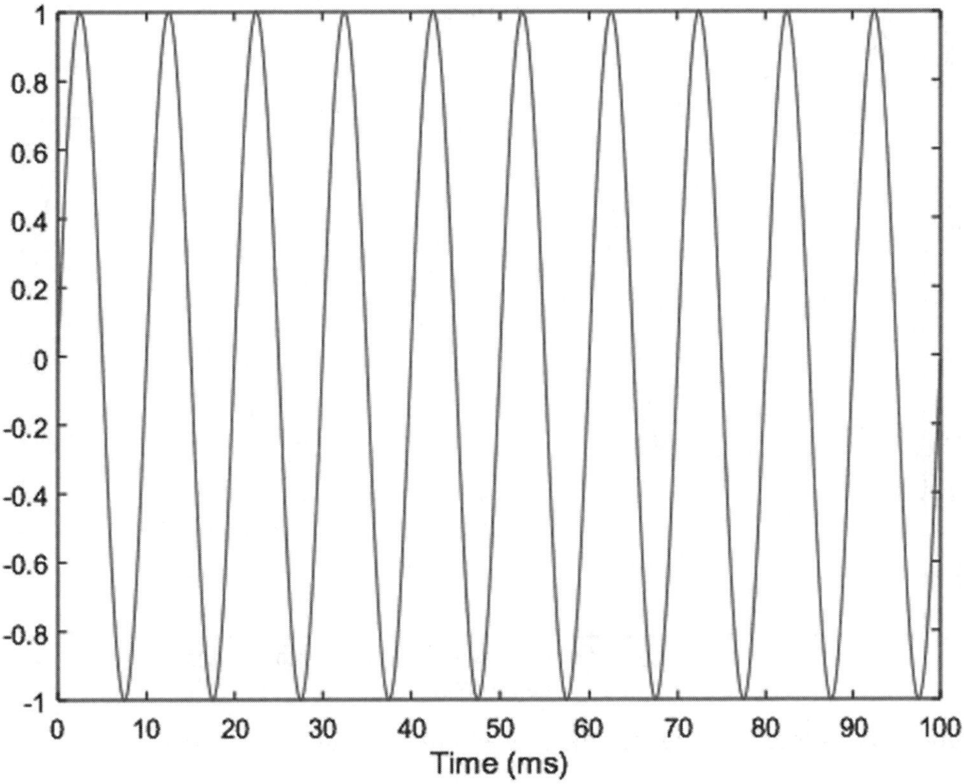

Figure 4–9. A simple 100-Hz sine tine.

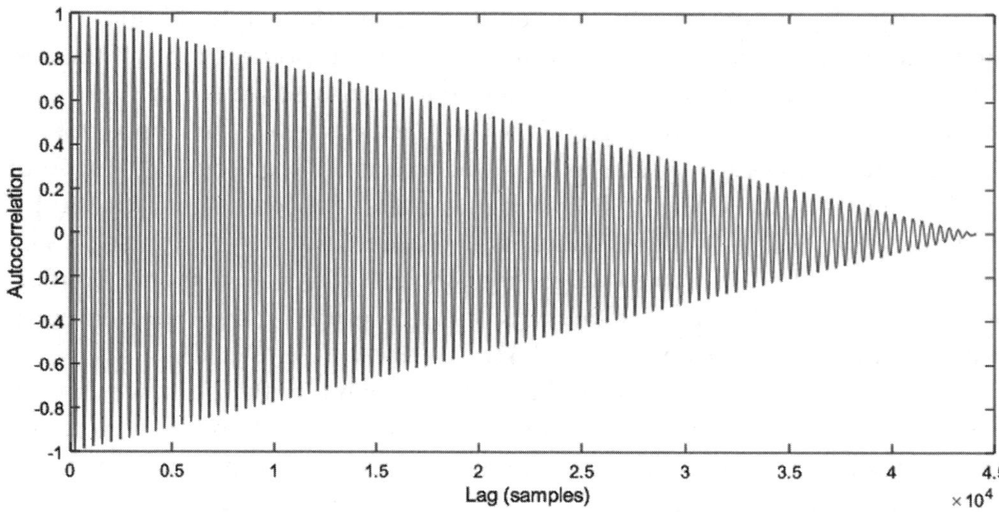

Figure 4–10. The corresponding autocorrelation sequence (nonnegative lags only).

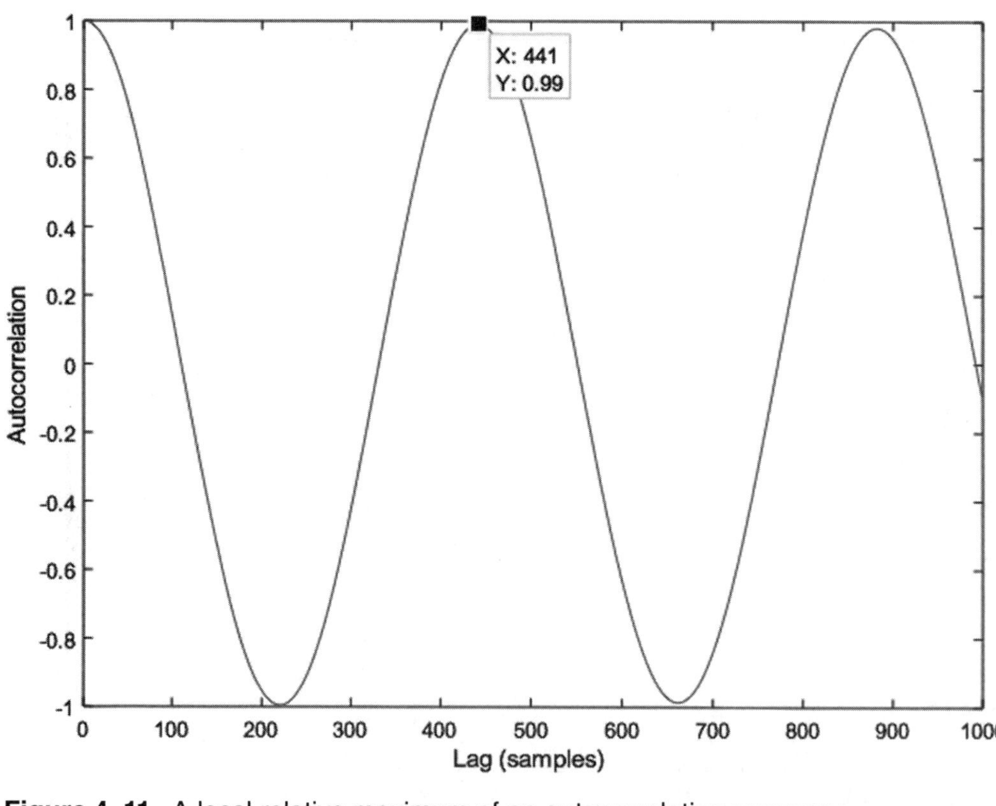

Figure 4–11. A local relative maximum of an autocorrelation sequence.

The same approach may be taken when analyzing vowels and other quasiperiodic waveforms (e.g., voiced fricatives, nasals, glides, and approximants), which can all carry pitch information.

Figure 4–12 shows a recording of the vowel /a/ and its corresponding autocorrelation sequence with lags converted into milliseconds, and a highlight on the first relative maximum. The autocorrelation sequence indicates a glottal pitch period of 7.313 ms, yielding an estimated pitch of approximately 137 Hz.

Listing 4–31 contains a MATLAB program to record a speaker's vowel and produce a similar plot indicating the estimated pitch. In this example, lag is converted into milliseconds to facilitate simple computation of glottal pitch period.

Listing 4–31. MATLAB routine to analyze a recorded vowel via autocorrelation

```
% Plot vowel data.
time = (1:length(y)) / fs;
subplot(2,1,1)
plot(time*1000, y)
xlabel('Time (ms)')
ylabel('Amplitude')

% Compute autocorrelation sequence.
[c, lags] = xcorr(y, 'coeff');

% Take only non-negative lag values.
c = c(lags >= 0);
lags = lags(lags >= 0);

% Convert lag to milliseconds.
lags_ms = lags / fs * 1000;

% Plot results.
subplot(2,1,2)
plot(lags_ms, c)
xlabel('Lag (ms)')
ylabel('Autocorrelation')
```

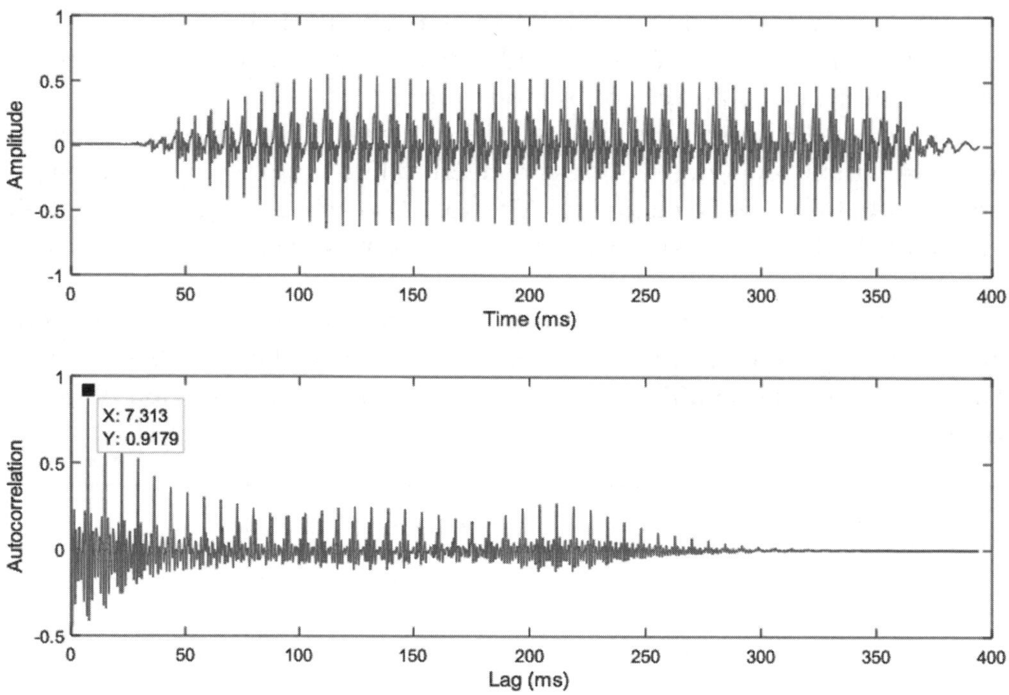

Figure 4–12. Waveform and autocorrelation sequence.

Just as it is possible to compute windowed spectra to arrive at a spectrogram, so too can one compute windowed autocorrelation sequences, extract the fundamental frequency, and arrive at a pitch track. Research in the field of pitch tracking has led to supplemental techniques as well, including leveraging spectral information and employing cepstral methods.

A variety of algorithms based on the above approaches exist, such as YAAPT (Zahorian & Hu, 2008), The Wu pitch-tracking system (Wu & Wang, 2002), and RAPT (Robust Algorithm for Pitch Tracking; Talkin, 1995), to name a few. This section will demonstrate usage of MATLAB routines for YAAPT (Figure 4–13); however, the steps are broadly similar for any given algorithm. Before the listing is run, the YAAPT files must be downloaded and added to the MATLAB path. It is assumed that the speech data have been recorded or imported into the variables `y` and `fs`. See Listing 4–32.

Listing 4–32. Usage of YAAPT

```
% Extract pitch using YAAPT.
% Note that frameLength is in milliseconds.
[pitch, nf, frameLength] = yaapt(y, fs, 1);
```

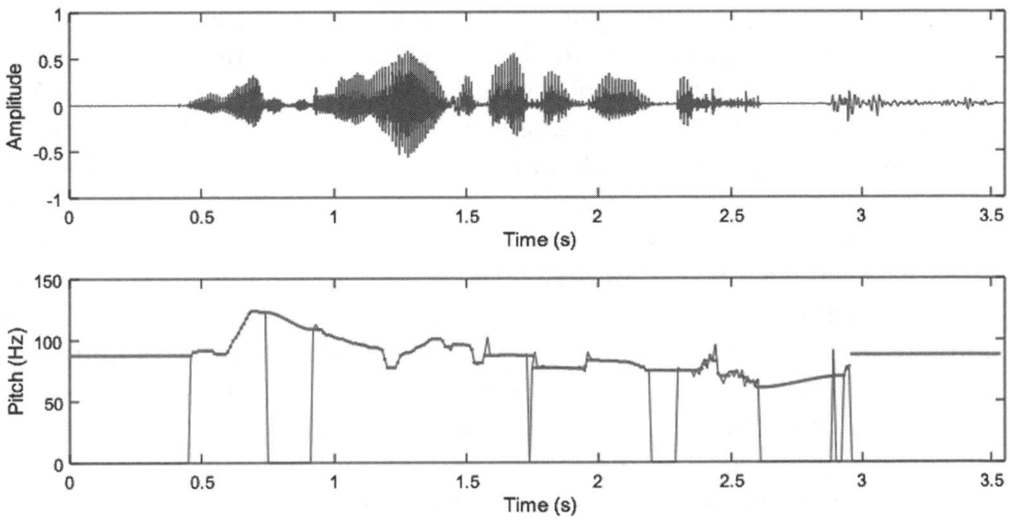

Figure 4–13. Example YAAPT output.

```
% Apply pitch fixing function to estimate pitch contours
% in voiceless regions.
pitch_fixed = ptch_fix(pitch);

% Plot original data.
subplot(2, 1, 1);
time = (1:length(y)) / fs;
plot(time, y)
maxTime = length(y) / fs;
xlim([0, maxTime])
xlabel('Time (s)')
ylabel('Amplitude')

% Plot pitch track.
subplot(2, 1, 2);
pitchTime = (1:length(pitch)) * fsp / 1000;
plot(pitchTime, pitch)
xlim([0, maxTime])
xlabel('Time (s)')
ylabel('Pitch (Hz)')

% Superimpose adjusted pitch track.
hold on
plot(pitchTime, pitch_fixed, '.', 'LineWidth', 2)
```

In Figure 4–13, the thick line represents the "fixed" pitch track, which attempts to estimate pitch contours for voiceless regions and supply a more continuous curve. This is particularly useful when fed into algorithms investigating the change in pitch over time in a given clinical task or experimental condition: the raw pitch track (thin line) often contains sharp discontinuities that can confound follow-up analyses. Rapid jumps in pitch, without correction and/or smoothing, may lead such analyses to report a higher pitch variation than is actually present. In particular, caution is recommended when the apparent pitch value jumps to twice or half its previous value. These types of jumps, as opposed to the ones that can be remedied through smoothing, are known as octave jumps, and must be corrected at the detection stage. Octave jumps occur when the pitch-tracking algorithm selects the wrong peak in the autocorrelation function (often due to missing the first peak). Fortunately, most modern algorithms such as YAAPT have inbuilt facilities for detecting and correcting for octave jumps before returning the pitch track to the user.

One must note, however, that such automated tracking tends to work best on passages with many voiced segments; these allow the patient ample opportunity to phonate. A preponderance of unvoiced segments, on the other hand, can confound pitch-tracking algorithms with multiple jump discontinuities.

Speech Rate Estimation for Diadochokinetic Tasks

In contrast to pitch tracking, speech rate estimation works best when all consonants are voiceless, since such passages admit the simplifying assumption that all voiced segments are vowels. In this case, the problem of detecting vocalic nuclei reduces to that of detecting voiced segments among unvoiced or silent sections of the recording. A clinical task to which this method is particularly suited is the computation of speech rate in diadochokinetic tasks (e.g., requesting the patient to produce repeated iterations of "pataka," "papapa," etc.).

Expanding on the code from earlier, we wish to count the number of voiced segments. Recall that voiced *samples* are indicated by a value of 2, whereas voiceless samples are indicated by a value of 1. Having modularized this task, we now take its output as input to a new algorithm that counts the transitions from 1 or 0 to 2 (voiceless or silent to voiced, indicating a vowel onset under our simplified passage structure). To do this, one could write a *for* loop that iterates through every sample of the recording and compares it to the previous one, but a better use of MATLAB's built-in vectorization is to do the computation in one or two steps, rather than the thousands of individual steps required by such a loop. We do this by forming a logical vector where `1` represents a vowel and `0` represents anything else. Then we take the difference of this vector using the `diff()` function. Whenever we transition *into* a vowel, this vector will have a value of 1; whenever a vowel ends, the vector will have a value of –1. We simply count the number of ones to estimate the number of vowels in the passage, and then divide by articulation time. See Listing 4–33.

Listing 4–33. Estimation of speech rate

```
% Compute the sample type for each sample in y.
sampleType = detectVoicing(y, fs);

% Count the number of times we transition into a vowel from anything else.
vowel = (sampleType == 2);
diffs = diff(vowel);
numVowels = sum(diffs == 1);

% Divide by articulation time to estimate articulation rate.
signalLength = length(y) / fs;
pauseSamples = sum(sampleType == 0);
pauseTime = pauseSamples / fs;
articTime = signalLength - pauseTime;
articRate = numVowels / articTime;
```

Measures of Speech Motor Control

Intrinsic and extrinsic prosody refer to two planning vectors along which speech is controlled systematically to accord with (a) the acoustics of a language and (b) the command aspects of communicative intent, respectively (Boutsen, 2008). Although the former vector pulls toward minimizing variability across identical utterances, the latter pulls toward increasing variability. Thus, if the communicative context and intent remain the same, it is to be expected that speakers control their utterances in a manner that achieves some degree of constancy or stability.

This idea of stability across utterances as an index of speech motor control has found conceptualization in the spatio-temporal index developed by Smith et al. (1995). Basically, this index is the summed variation over repeated (at least eight) utterances seen within a moving window that is sliding across time-normalized metrics, such as oral aperture or lip distance, from the beginning to end. The now classic utterance used for this measurement is the phrase "Buy Bobby a puppy," repeated eight times. The index is spatial in that it is obtained from the lip/jaw kinematics that effect an open closing cycle across the CV CVCV V CVCV sequence. Ideal repetitions of the utterance (i.e., exact copies) would produce the same "wave"; if overlaid on each other, the plot would show 1 wave covering the other ones behind or below. If we were to compare the waves, say, for eight ideal, identical repetitions by dividing the normalized time interval from 0 to 1 into 50 points and summing the standard deviations for each from the beginning to the end each point would yield a standard deviation of zero, leading to a total of zero (Figure 4–14).

Of course, this is not what is observed in speech. Even simple utterances cannot be controlled perfectly. Furthermore, it appears that complexities introduced by the language, such as addenda to the "Buy Bobby a puppy" sequence generated by adding length and grammatical complexity (e.g., "Buy Bobby a puppy if he wants one"), result in greater kinematic variability even when just considering the original sequence extracted from the whole.

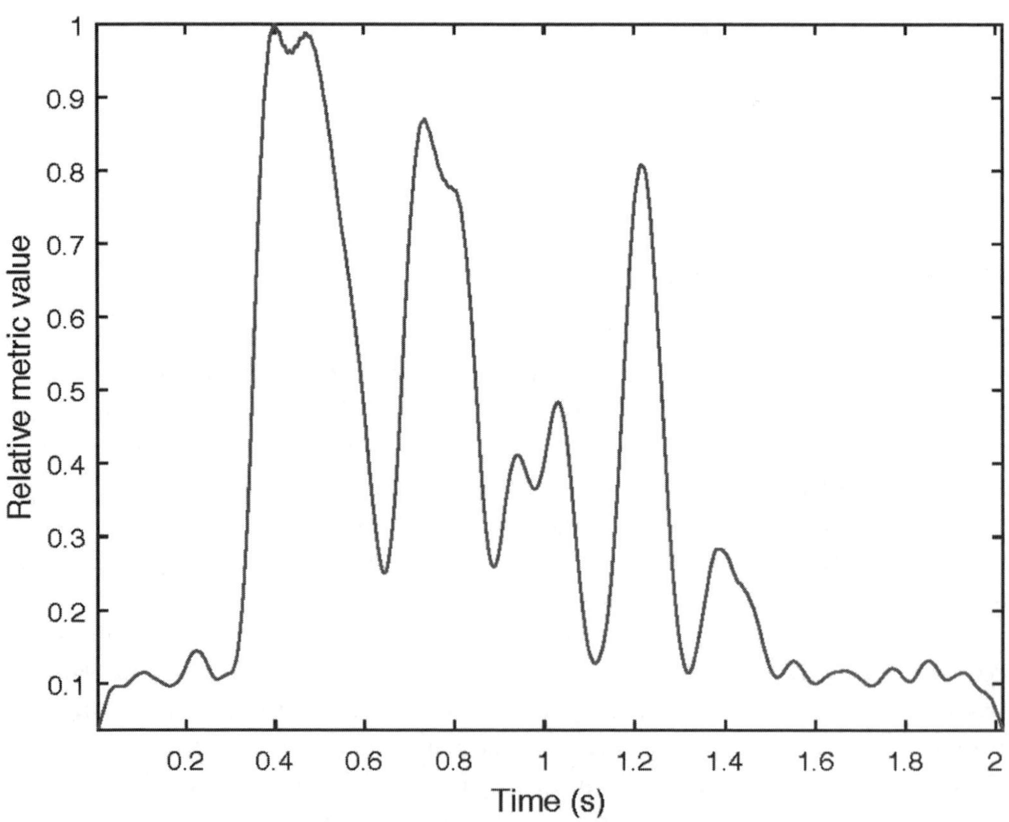

Figure 4–14. An example of identical signals.

The spatio-temporal index, while novel in its own right, also introduced MATLAB to the speech pathology community as the magic behind its computation. In what follows we will try to dispel some of that magic and detail how this measure is derived. More recently, some investigators (Boutsen, Deweber, & Dvorak, 2011; Howell, Anderson, Bartrip, & Bailey, 2009) have considered deriving an acoustic temporal index, which is based on amplitude envelopes rather than kinematic measures. Typically, the amplitude envelopes are computed from the onset of the first consonant (/b/) to the offset of voicing of the final vowel (/i/) (Howell et al., 2009). They are then time-normalized and compared in a similar fashion as are the kinematic signals. Obtaining this index is less intrusive and also less expensive since it does not require face-tracking equipment. We will conclude by illustrating the ATI alternative to the STI.

Algorithmically, computation of the STI, ATI, or any similar measure can be divided into four steps: data input and preprocessing, extraction of the metric waveform (e.g., kinematic or amplitude envelope), time normalization, and computation of variability.

The first step has been extensively covered in this chapter, so will not be elaborated on here. We begin by assuming that the data already exist in some set of variables, have undergone filtering or noise removal, and have been properly trimmed to the extent of the word.

The second step may involve envelope extraction (e.g., Hilbert envelope) for acoustic data and/or smoothing of kinematic data, depending on the measure selected. Smoothing, as covered above, can be performed by convolving the raw signal with a column vector of weights, termed the kernel. Typically, kernels are normalized, meaning that the sum of all elements in the kernel is constrained. To effect a weighted average, kernels are normalized to 1.

The third step involves resampling all signals onto the interval (0, 1). Assuming the onset and offset points of each signal are marked in the preprocessing step, the resampling will map the beginning of the signal to time 0 and the end to time 1 (Figure 4–15).

In MATLAB, this resampling can be most readily accomplished by `interp1` function, which is used for one-dimensional interpolation. Although the `resample` function, given its name, would seem more appropriate, `interp1` provides an easy way to specify the points required for analysis. For the following code (Listing 4–34), assume that the signal of interest is passed to the function in the variable `y`, and that `nPoints` is some integer greater than 1. Note that sampling rate information is not needed, since (a) all signals from the same patient should have the same sampling rate, having been recorded with the same equipment, and (b) any signals with a higher sampling rate will be normalized to the same "rate" of 50 samples per 1 normalized time unit anyway. Also, for later computational purposes, the vector of indices is transposed to form a column vector, rather than row vector.

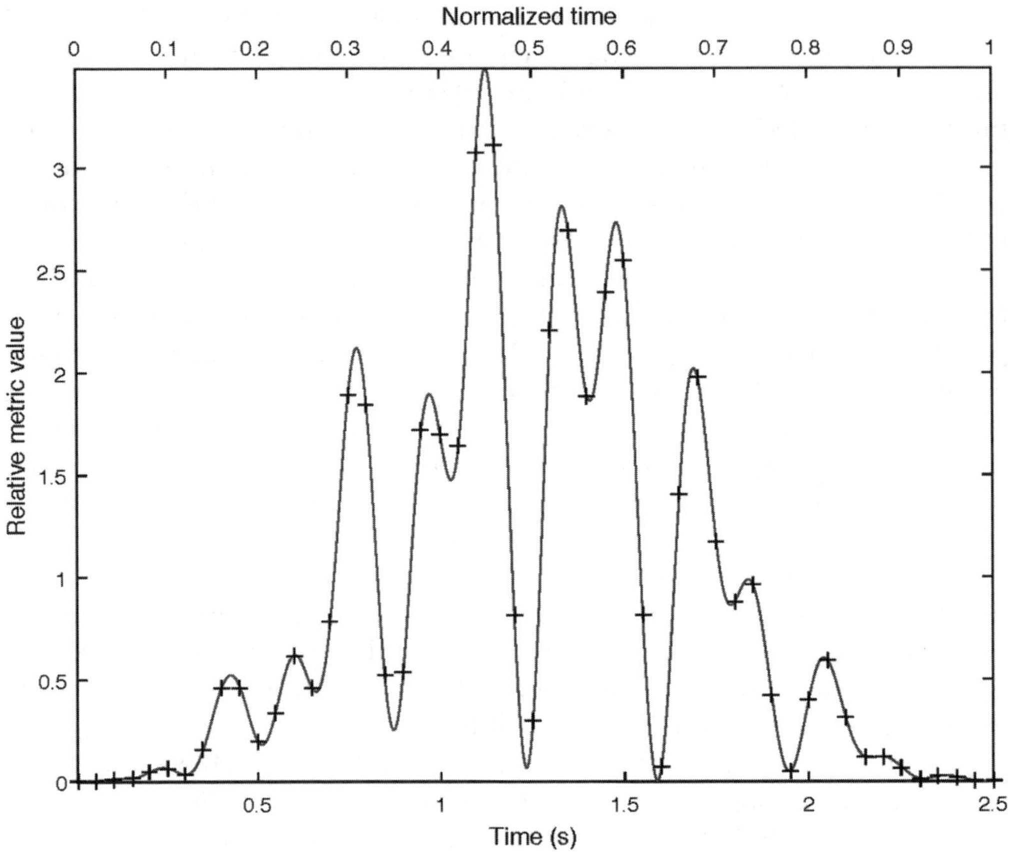

Figure 4–15. Time normalization through resampling.

Listing 4–34. Time-normalization

```
function y = timenormalize(y, nPoints)

    % Compute points to interpolate. These are index values.
    indices = linspace(1, length(y), nPoints)';

    % Interpolate y on the specified indices.
    y = interp1(1:length(y), y, indices);

end
```

The final step then requires computation of the sum of standard deviations at each interpolated point. We assume that all signals will be of different lengths at the outset. One way to store them is in a cell array of column vectors; a matrix, for example, would require equal lengths in samples. Suppose we load the signals in as follows (Listing 4–35).

Listing 4–35. Loading files into a cell array

```
% Load audio files into a cell array.
Y = cell(1, 10);
Y{1} = audioread('patient 1-1.wav');
Y{2} = audioread('patient 1-2.wav');
% ...
Y{10} = audioread('patient 1-10.wav');
```

We can then iterate through each one and normalize it with the above function (Listing 4–36). Importantly, this will lead to a cell array of equally long column vectors.

Listing 4–36. Iteration and normalization

```
for i = 1:10
    % Perform filtering or smoothing here.
    % ...

    % Time normalize.
    Y{i} = timenormalize(Y{i}, nPoints);

end
```

After this, we can use the `cell2mat` function to create a 50-by-*n* matrix from the normalized signals. The transpose operator is used again to convert this to a *n*-by-50 matrix. Finally, we compute the vector sum of the columnwise standard deviations (Listing 4–37).

Listing 4–37. Transposition and computation of index

```
% Convert to a matrix and orient for columnwise computation.
Y = cell2mat(Y)';

% Compute index.
index = sum(std(Y));
```

Exercises

1. Rewrite the importing code in Listing 4–35 to be less repetitive. Hint: Consider using the `uigetfile()` function with `'multiselect'` set to `'on'`.
2. Combine the above code into a single function that accepts a cell array of files as its input argument and returns the associated acoustic temporal index. If the user does not specify the files, the function should bring up a dialog box to allow him/her to select them. Be sure to code for contingencies (canceled dialog box, invalid files, etc.)!
3. (Advanced) Notice that the above algorithm requires importing all of the audio files into a large matrix. Suppose we were working with a long passage, or had a large number of files, possibly leading to exorbitant memory usage and/or poor performance. How might we divide the computation into smaller blocks? *Hint: Consider cumulatively updating the standard deviations as additional files are read in.*

References

American Speech-Language-Hearing Association. (2004). *Preferred practice patterns for the profession of speech-language pathology*. Retrieved from http://www.asha.org/policy/PP2004-00191/

Beck, D. L., & Nilsson, M. (2013, May). Speech-in-noise testing: A pragmatic addendum to hearing aid fittings. *Hearing Review*.

Bohland, J. W., Bullock, D., & Guenther, F. H. (2010). Neural representations and mechanisms for the performance of simple speech sequences. *Journal of Cognitive Neuroscience*, *7*, 1504, 1529.

Boutsen, F. R., Deweber, D. D., & Dvorak, J. D. (2011). Intrinsic and extrinsic prosody control in normal speakers. *Stem-, Spraak- en Taalpathologie*, *17*(S), 87.

Brookes, M. (2013). Voicebox: Speech processing toolbox for MATLAB [Computer software]. Version 2803. Retrieved from http://www.ee.ic.ac.uk/hp/staff/dmb/voicebox/voicebox.html

Butterworth, S. (1930). On the theory of filter amplifiers. *Wireless Engineer*, *7*, 536–541.

Colton, R. H., & Casper, J. K. (2011). *Understanding voice problems: A physiological perspective for diagnosis and treatment* (4th ed.). Baltimore, MD: Lippincott Williams & Wilkins.

Darley, F. L., Aronson, A. E., & Brown, J. R. (1975). *Motor speech disorders* (3rd ed.). Philadelphia, PA: W. B. Saunders.

Dunn, L. M., & Dunn, D. M. (2007). *Peabody Picture Vocabulary Test* (4th ed.). San Antonio, TX: Pearson.

Ellis, D. P. W. (2004). Sinewave speech analysis/synthesis in MATLAB. Retrieved from http://labrosa.ee.columbia.edu/matlab/sws/

Fant, G. (1960). *Acoustic theory of speech perception*. The Hague, Netherlands: Mouton & Co.

Fillinger, A. (2008). *The NIST speech SNR measurement*. Retrieved from http://www.nist.gov/smartspace/nist_speech_snr_measurement.html

Frear, M. (2004). MATLAB multi-channel audio, v 0.2 [Computer program]. Retrieved from http://www.mathworks.com/matlabcentral/fileexchange/4017-pa-wavplay

Fujisaki, H., & Hirose, K. (1984). Analysis of voice fundamental frequency contours for declarative sentences of Japanese. *Journal of the Acoustical Society of Japan, 5*(4), 233–241.

Goldman, R., & Fristoe, M. (2000). *Goldman-Fristoe Test of Articulation 2*. San Antonio, TX: Pearson.

Goldman, R., Fristoe, M. W., & Woodcock, R. W. (1971). A new dimension in the assessment of speech sound discrimination. *Journal of Learning Disabilities, 4*(7), 364.

Grosjean, F. (1980). Spoken word recognition processes and the gating paradigm. *Perception & Psychophysics, 28*(4), 267–283.

Guenther, F. H. (1994). A neural network model of speech acquisition and motor equivalent speech production. *Biological Cybernetics, 72*, 43–53.

Guenther, F. H., Brumberg, J. S., Wright, E. J., Nieto-Castanon, A., Tourville, J. A., Panko, M., . . . Kennedy, P. R. (2009). A wireless brain-machine interface for real-time speech synthesis. *PLoS One, 4*(12), e8218.

Guenther, F. H., Ghosh, S. S., & Tourville, J. A. (2006). Neural modeling and imaging of the cortical interactions underlying syllable production. *Brain and Language, 96*, 280–301.

Hervais-Adelman, A., Pefkou, M., & Golestani, N. (2014). Bilingual speech-in-noise: Neural bases of semantic context use in the native language. *Brain and Language, 132*, 1–6.

Hilbert, D. (1953). *Grundzüge einer allgemeinen Theorie der linearen Integralgleichungen*. Providence, RI: Chelsea.

Howell, P., Anderson, A. J., Bartrip, J., & Bailey, E. (2009). Comparison of acoustic and kinematic approaches to measuring utterance-level speech variability. *Journal of Speech, Language, and Hearing Research, 52*(4), 1088–1096.

Jenkins, J. J., & Strange, W. (1999). Perception of dynamic information for vowels in syllable onsets and offsets. *Perception & Psychophysics, 61*(6), 1200–1210.

Kalveram, K. T. (1991). How pathological autio-phonatoric coupling induces stuttering: A model of speech flow control. In H. F. M. Peters, W. Hulstijn, & C. W. Starkweather (Eds.), *Speech motor control and stuttering: Proceedings of the 2nd International Conference on Speech Motor Control and Stuttering* (pp. 163–170). Amsterdam, Netherlands: Excerpta Media.

Karam, M., Khazaal, H. F., Aglan, H., & Cole, C. (2014). Noise removal in speech processing using spectral subtraction. *Journal of Signal and Information Processing, 5*, 32–41.

Kent, R. D., & Read, C. (1992). *The acoustic analysis of speech*. San Diego, CA: Singular.

Kent, R. D., & Rosenbek, J. C. (1983). Acoustic patterns of apraxia of speech. *Journal of Speech and Hearing Research*, *26*(2), 231–249.

Kertesz, A. (2006). *Western Aphasia Battery-Revised*. San Antonio, TX: Pearson.

Klatt, D. H. (1980). Software for a cascade/parallel formant synthesizer. *Journal of the Acoustical Society of America*, *67*(3), 971–995.

Ladefoged, P. (1996). *Elements of acoustic phonetics*. Chicago, IL: University of Chicago Press.

Lindfield, K. C., Wingfield, A., & Goodglass, H. (1999). The contribution of prosody to spoken word recognition. *Applied Psycholinguistics*, *20*, 395–405.

Maeda, S. (1988). Improved articulatory model. *Journal of the Acoustical Society of America*, *84*(Suppl. 1), S146.

McLennan, S. (2000). *Klatt synthesizer in Simulink®*. Retrieved from http://www.shaav.com/professional/linguistics/klatt.pdf.

Mixdorff, H. (2000). A novel approach to fully automatic extraction of Fujisaki model parameters. *Proceedings ICASSP 2000*, *3*, 1281–1284.

Nilsson, M., Soli, S. D., & Sullivan, J. A. (1994). Development of the Hearing in Noise Test for the measurement of speech reception thresholds in quiet and in noise. *Journal of the Acoustical Society of America*, *95*(2), 1085–1099.

O'Shaughnessy, D. (1988). Linear predictive coding. *IEEE Potentials*, *7*(1), 29–32.

Patel, R., & Campellone, P. (2009). Acoustic and perceptual cues to contrastive stress in dysarthria. *Journal of Speech, Language, and Hearing Research*, *52*, 206–222.

Pierrehumbert, J. (1980). *The phonology and phonetics of English intonation* (Doctoral dissertation). MIT, Cambridge, MA.

Quantieri, T. F. (2001). *Discrete-time speech signal processing: Principles and practice*. Upper Saddle River, NJ: Prentice Hall.

Remez, R. E., Rubin, P. E., Pisoni, D. B., & Carrel, T. D. (1981). Speech perception without traditional speech cues. *Science*, *212*, 947–950.

Rogers, C. L., & Lopez, A. S. (2008). Perception of silent-center syllables by native and non-native English speakers. *Journal of the Acoustical Society of America*, *124*(2), 1278–1293.

Rubin, P. E. (1980). *Sinewave synthesis* [Internal memo]. New Haven, CT: Haskins Laboratories.

Rubin, P. E., Ellis, D., & Frost, S. (1996). Sinewave synthesis [MATLAB code]. New Haven, CT: Haskins Laboratories.

Silverman, K., Beckman, M., Pitrelli, J., Ostendorf, M., Pierrehumbert, J., Hirschberg, J., & Price, P. (1992, October). TOBI: A Standard Scheme for Labeling Prosody. In J. Ohala (Ed.), *Proceedings of the 2nd International Conference on Spoken Language Processing 92* (pp. 867–870). Edmonton, AB: University of Alberta.

Smith, A., Goffman, L., Zelaznik, H. N., Ying, G., & McGillem, C. (1995). Spatiotemporal stability and patterning of speech movement sequences. *Experimental Brain Research*, *104*(3), 493–501.

Smith, S. W. (2002). *Digital signal processing: A practical guide for engineers and scientists*. Burlington, MA: Elsevier Science.

Snell, R. C., & Milinazzo, F. (1993). Formant location from LPC analysis data. *IEEE® Transactions on Speech and Audio Processing, 1*(2), 129–134.

Song, J. H., Skoe, E., Banai, K., & Kraus, N. (2012). Training to improve hearing speech in noise: Biological mechanism. *Cerebral Cortex, 22*, 1180–1190.

Stellars, C., Stanton, A. E., McConnachie, A., Dunnet, C. P., Chapman, L. M., Bucknall, C. E., & MacKenzie, K. (2009). Reliability of perceptions of voice quality: Evidence from a problem asthma clinic population. *Journal of Laryngology and Otology, 123*(7), 755–763.

Stevens, K. M. (2000). *Acoustic phonetics*. Cambridge, MA: MIT Press.

Strange, W., Jenkins, J. J., & Johnson, T. L. (1983). Dynamic specification of coarticulated vowels. *Journal of the Acoustical Society of America, 74*, 695–705.

Talkin, D. (1995). A robust algorithm for pitch tracking (RAPT). In W. B. Kleijn & K. K. Paliwal (Eds.), *Speech coding and synthesis* (pp. 495–518). Amsterdam, Netherlands: Elsevier Science.

Titze, I. R. (1994). *Principles of voice production*. Englewood Cliffs, NJ: Prentice-Hall.

Van Riper, C. (1963). *Speech correction* (4th ed.). Englewood Cliffs, NJ: Prentice-Hall.

Von Hapsburg, D., & Bahng, J. (2009). Effects of noise on bilingual listeners' first language (L1) speech perception. *Perspectives on Hearing and Hearing Disorders: Research and Diagnostics, 13*, 21–26.

Wu, M., & Wang, D. L. (2002). *A multi-pitch tracking algorithm for noisy speech*. Paper presented at the 2002 IEEE International Conference on Acoustics, Speech, and Signal Processing (ICASSP), Orlando, FL.

Zahorian, S. A., & Hu, H. (2008). A spectral/temporal method for robust fundamental frequency tracking. *Journal of the Acoustical Society of America, 123*, 4559–4571.

5

Clinic Data Management and Analysis

Electronic Medical Records: A Brief Introduction

Electronic medical records (EMRs), also known as electronic health records, are organized databases of clinical or demographic information about a clinic's patients (Gunter & Terry, 2005). EMRs have gained in popularity in recent decades, with promises of greater productivity, better clinical management, and improved patient care. However, not all practices benefit from the introduction of what can often be an expensive investment (Himmelstein, Wright, & Woolhandler, 2010). In fact, for single-clinician offices or smaller practices (particularly as seen in speech-language pathology [SLP] and audiology), the number of patients seen may not meet the threshold for cost-effectiveness of "turnkey" systems designed for larger institutions (Congressional Budget Office [CBO], 2008).

This is not to say that EMRs are to be avoided in SLP and audiology practices. Costs aside, properly implemented EMRs have been shown to improve patient care (Cebul, Love, Jain, & Hebert, 2011) and improve efficiency (Liu & Nicholas, 2009). Furthermore, such systems facilitate clinical knowledge discovery and data mining (e.g., Fayyad, Piatetsky-Shapiro, & Smyth, 1996; Frawley, Piatetsky-Shapiro, & Matheus, 1992), which can uncover important trends in patient data and lead to improved clinical decision making. However, given the unique patient base of most speech and audiology clinics, the entry of data into a stationary computer system is infeasible, and the required mobility of providers can be a barrier to computerization. In traditional clinical settings, this has led providers to continue to rely on pen-and-paper methods, which can slow or even prevent data entry (Cleophas & Zwinderman, 2015) and subsequent mining.

What is needed is an open standard that connects commonly used speech and hearing assessments and tools in a digital format to a centralized, secure database system. Such a standard would (a) allow for in-room data capture on mobile devices such as tablets, laptop computers, and smartphones (Broughton, Lashlee, Marcum, & Mustata-Wilson, 2013); (b) comply with **Health Insurance Portability and Accountability Act** (HIPAA) and other relevant legislation to ensure confidentiality and security of patient data; and (c) facilitate secured transmission of the gathered data to a centralized database or event aggregation server. After aggregation, clinicians can generate reports to evaluate efficacy, patient progress, provider efficiency, and many other useful clinical metrics.

Although we do not propose the following example as a unifying standard across all of health care, it serves as a useful model for small-scale, individualized software development that can be tailored to the needs of a specific clinic or patient population. Specifically, the clinical scenario presented in this chapter focuses on the final aspect of the desired system: the generation of reports and extraction of useful information.

Data Organization in MATLAB® With Tables

Before delving into the specifics of our example implementation, it is useful to outline the most common methods for organizing data in MATLAB. In advance, we know that clinical data sets will be heterogeneous, in that they will contain a variety of different data types. For example, patient names and identifiers (e.g., clinic ID numbers) will likely be stored as strings of characters, whereas test scores will be stored as integers or floating-point values. Furthermore, rich data such as audio recordings may also be collected and stored for later analysis.

We have previously covered the concept of a structure, which allows one to store heterogeneous data for a single instance of an abstract object, be it a patient, a test score, or a clinical visit. However, when seeking to organize data for knowledge discovery, it is important to ensure compatibility between observations, which could be violated by using only structures. This compatibility can be achieved by using a `table` object instead.

Tables are a MATLAB-internal way to organize column-oriented data. Columns indicate different variables or properties of interest, whereas rows indicate observations. In our example, each column will refer to an aspect of a patient-contact session. Separate columns will be used to store the patient's ID number, the clinician's ID number, the date and time of the session, as well as the results of the session. Each row will indicate a single session. A single patient may therefore have multiple rows, allowing clinicians to track progress over time.

Tables can be created with the `table` command, and combine data from the Workspace into a single object. For example, suppose we have the following code that produces the two columns (note the transpose operator) `x` and `y`, then combines them into a table:

```
>> x = (1:10)';
>> y = x.^2;
>> t = table(x, y);
```

This will create a table object (Figure 5–1) with two columns labeled "x" and "y."

```
>> t

t =

     x      y
    ___    ___

     1       1
     2       4
     3       9
     4      16
     5      25
     6      36
     7      49
     8      64
     9      81
    10     100
```

Figure 5–1. An example of a `table` object.

Because both of these variables are doubles (i.e., numeric), the `summary` function gives useful information (Figure 5–2) about them when applied to the table object `t`:

```
>> summary(t)
```

Common database operations are also available for table objects. For example, the functions `innerjoin` and `outerjoin` perform inner and outer joins, respectively. An inner join is one in which only records common to both tables are returned. Outer joins come in three types: left outer joins, right outer joins, and full outer joins. Left and right joins return the same records as an inner join, plus additional records from the first or second table, respectively, that do not match the opposite table. Full outer joins simply combine all data from both tables into a single, large table. In both cases, missing values may exist when the variables on which the join is performed (e.g., the key variables) do not have the same set of values in both tables.

In a clinical setting, join operations are most commonly used to merge, for example, a table with patient characteristics and demographics and a

```
>> summary(t)

Variables:

    x: 10x1 double
        Values:

            min          1
            median     5.5
            max         10

    y: 10x1 double
        Values:

            min            1
            median      30.5
            max          100
```

Figure 5–2. Typical output from the `summary` function.

table of encounters, so that the resultant table allows stratification and comparison of outcomes by patient characteristics. For example, one might want to use such commands to examine the progress made by patients with autism spectrum disorder (ASD) under a given therapy protocol as compared to neurotypical patients, while not requiring the clinician to record each patient's ASD status at every interaction. In performing joins, it is necessary to specify key variables, which are used to match records. For clinical data, patient IDs are common key variables, as they allow linkage of data while preserving anonymity (so long as the "contact" or "billing" tables, for example, remain excluded).

In Listing 5–1, we demonstrate the creation and joining of two tables, denoted `records` and `patients`. We use the `innerjoin` function to avoid selecting patients who do not have any clinical session records (as may occur if a report is run before the session is completed, but after an appointment is made and the patient's information entered into the system). We also wish to avoid selecting session records for which the corresponding patient's demographic information does not exist. In a properly designed EMR system, this should not occur, but using an inner join ensures that the retrieved data table contains the proper observations. The `records` table exemplifies the type of data that would be recorded over several clinical sessions for a small patient pool. The `patients` table contains typical demographic information. One item of note is that, while "age" may be considered demographic, the typical span of speech and hearing services over childhood can often involve several years of data. Therefore, the MATLAB `datetime` type is used to indicate the patient's date of birth and is compared with additional `datetime` data for date of service to compute the patient's age at each treatment session. An additional important syntactic detail is the use of semicolons rather than commas to separate elements of arrays. This is because the `table` function requires its input variables to be column arrays.

Listing 5–1. Creating sample patient and clinical data

```
% Example patient data.
id = {'123'; '456'; '789'};
dob = [datetime(2000, 01, 01); ...
    datetime(2010, 04, 08); ...
    datetime(2007, 12, 15)];
gender = {'M'; 'F'; 'F'};
patients = table(id, dob, gender, ...
    'VariableNames', {'PatientID', 'DoB', 'Gender'});
```

```
% Example (weekly) treatment data.
id = {'123'; '123'; '456'; '123'; '789'};
date = [datetime(2015, 01, 15); ...
    datetime(2015, 01, 22); ...
    datetime(2015, 01, 22); ...
    datetime(2015, 01, 29); ...
    datetime(2015, 01, 29)];
score = [75; 78; 60; 81; 90];
records = table(id, date, score, ...
    'VariableNames', {'PatientID', 'DoS', 'TestScore'});

% Merge.
data = innerjoin(records, patients, 'Keys', 'PatientID');
```

The results of this operation are presented in Figure 5–3.

Although not demonstrated here, it is possible to join tables even if the ID variable is named something different in both. This can be done through the `LeftKeys` and `RightKeys` parameters in the `innerjoin` function.

A useful operation to perform on the new, joined data set might be to examine a patient's test score over time or by age. To compute a patient's age from date data, one can subtract the `DoB` field from the `DoS` field to determine a date difference. This is done with the `between` function, which returns an object of type `calendarDuration`, applied to the two fields. Just as with structures, table fields are accessed with the dot operator (`.`).

In Listing 5–2, we wish to determine the patient's age in years (with decimal fraction). This is done with the `split` function, followed by making an appropriate combination of the output arguments. The `split` function

```
>> data

data =

    PatientID        DoB          Gender        DoS          TestScore
    _________    ___________    ______    ___________    _________

    '123'        01-Jan-2000    'M'       15-Jan-2015    75
    '123'        01-Jan-2000    'M'       22-Jan-2015    78
    '123'        01-Jan-2000    'M'       29-Jan-2015    81
    '456'        08-Apr-2010    'F'       22-Jan-2015    60
    '789'        15-Dec-2007    'F'       29-Jan-2015    90
```

Figure 5–3. Creating a table from variables in the Workspace.

returns one output argument for each interval type requested (e.g., years, months, and days), so we combine these together to estimate years (using an approximate value of 365.25 days per year to account for leap years).

Listing 5–2. Computing patient age

```
% Exctract age at session.
data.Age = between(data.DoB, data.DoS);

% Convert duration to years.
[y, m, d] = split(data.Age, {'years', 'months', 'days'});
data.Age = y + m/12 + d/365.25;
```

The result of this computation is demonstrated in Figure 5–4.

In this example, we have the greatest amount of data on patient number 123. Suppose we wish to plot this patient's test score by his age (Listing 5–3). To do this, we need to subset the data so that only records from this patient are examined. This involves creating a Boolean expression to indicate which rows we want. In this case, we want only the rows in which the patient ID is equal to the string `'123'`, so we use the `strcmp` function. The results of this plot are illustrated in Figure 5–5, which suggests patient improvement over the course of several sessions.

Listing 5–3. Extracting information for a single patient

```
% Get info on patient 123.
rows = strcmp(data.PatientID, '123');
pt123data = data(rows, {'Age', 'TestScore'});
```

```
>> data

data =

    PatientID        DoB          Gender        DoS          TestScore        age
    _________    ___________    ______    ___________    _________    ___________

    '123'        01-Jan-2000    'M'       15-Jan-2015    75               15y 14d
    '123'        01-Jan-2000    'M'       22-Jan-2015    78               15y 21d
    '123'        01-Jan-2000    'M'       29-Jan-2015    81               15y 28d
    '456'        08-Apr-2010    'F'       22-Jan-2015    60           4y 9mo 14d
    '789'        15-Dec-2007    'F'       29-Jan-2015    90           7y 1mo 14d
```

Figure 5–4. Using `table` objects to store derived variables.

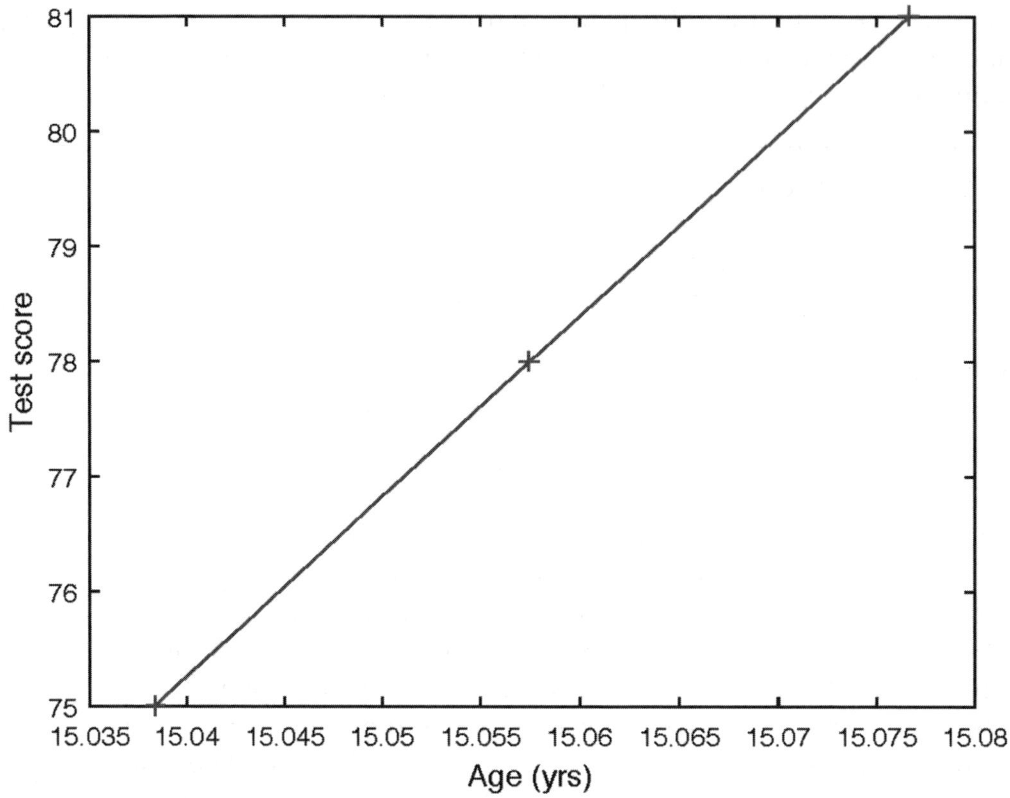

Figure 5–5. Generation of plots from `table` objects.

```
% Plot test score by age.
plot(pt123data.Age, pt123data.TestScore);
xlabel('Age (yrs)')
ylabel('Test score')
```

We can also plot test score by session number. This could be useful if we were interested in, say, the mean number of sessions a patient requires before reaching a certain level of improvement. In this case, it is actually easier than plotting by date (assuming proper sorting), since the index position of the test score will correspond to the session number (Figure 5–6).

Suppose that, for any of a variety of reasons, the data in the session table are **not** sorted in ascending date order, and we wish to organize the data by date, within patient. This can be accomplished with the `sortrows` function:

```
>> data = sortrows(data, {'PatientID', 'DoS'});
```

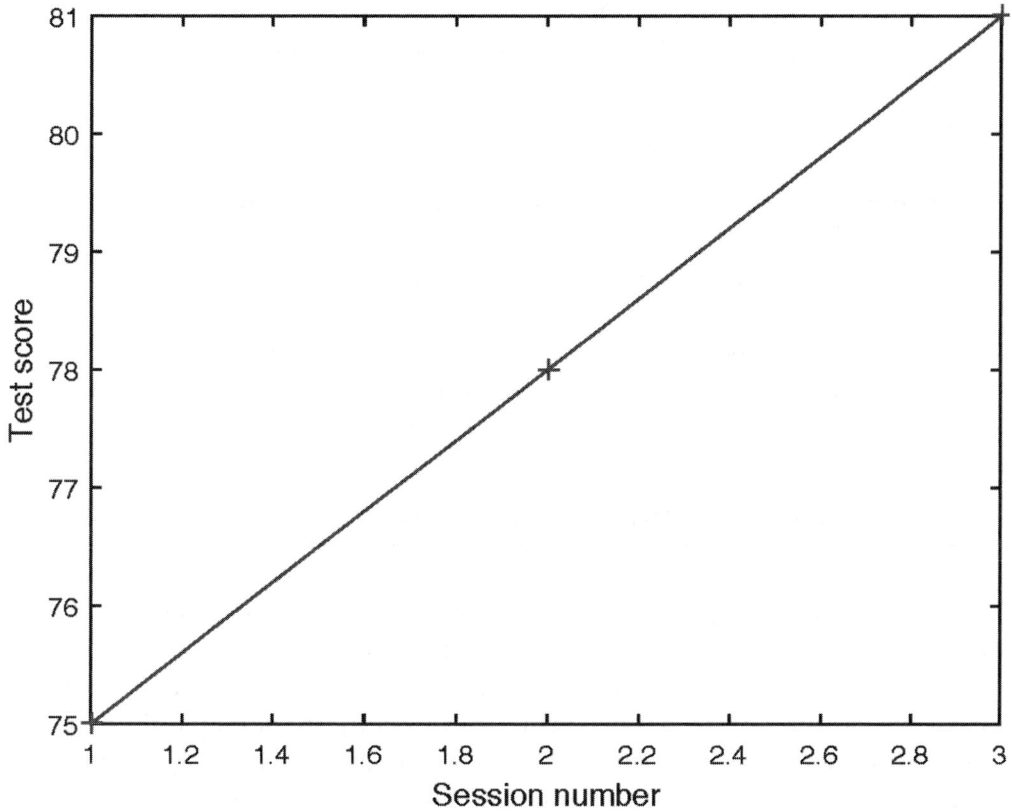

Figure 5–6. Plotting test score by session number.

Storage and Retrieval of Tables

Like many other types of data in MATLAB, table objects can be saved to and loaded from files on disk. The key functions for these operations are `writetable` and `readtable`, respectively.

The `writetable` function allows one to export tables into a variety of well-known data interchange formats, such as comma-separated value files (`.csv`), tab-delimited text files (`.txt`), or Excel spreadsheets (`.xls` or `.xlsx`). Situations in which one might want to export a table include exchanging data with colleagues, saving a record of patients and sessions for backup purposes, or integrating MATLAB into an existing workflow that relies on these formats. For example, one might have statistical analysis routines already prepared in SAS or R, and simply wish to export clinical data gathered in a MATLAB table object to those environments for modeling and analysis.

The following command demonstrates the export of the complete clinical data set example, including the derived age variable:

```
>> writetable(data, 'clinicData.xlsx');
```

Reading a table is just as simple, and proceeds as follows:

```
>> data = readtable('clinicData.xlsx');
```

This command reads the data stored in the file myClinicData.xlsx in the current directory and creates a corresponding table object in the Workspace.

Data Mining and Knowledge Discovery

Data mining, to a rough approximation, is the process of extracting information from a collection of data for the purposes of generating useful knowledge, or performing knowledge discovery. Bramer (2013) defines knowledge discovery as "the non-trivial extraction of implicit, previously unknown and potentially useful information from data." There are two main applications of data mining in which a clinician or clinic manager may be interested: description and prediction.

In descriptive data mining, one aims to describe some aspect of a clinic or practice in a quantitative way. For example, a useful application would be to describe the demographics of one's patient population in terms of age, ethnicity, gender, insurance status, and so on. Such a summary could provide valuable information to clinic managers.

In predictive data mining, the goal is to infer patterns from the existing data, which are used in turn to predict outcomes or trends for new patients. For example, suppose we wish to evaluate the in-clinic efficacy of a certain treatment program in terms of time-to-achievement for a particular goal. Under certain assumptions, this could be predicted by constructing a mathematical model of time to achievement in terms of relevant factors, such as age, comorbidities, initial ability level, and so on. Then, given a new patient, one could use this model to estimate the number of treatment sessions to schedule.

Another use of predictive data mining is in assessing cost-effectiveness. By merging billing information with session data, a clinic manager could determine which treatment programs achieve a better improvement to money/time ratio, adjusted for demographics.

A Clinical Scenario

For the remainder of this chapter, we explore a data-mining and analysis scenario for a hypothetical, small speech and hearing clinic. This clinic is targeted at elementary-school-age children (approximately 4 to 12 years of age) and provides a 16-week therapy program, corresponding to a semester at a tertiary or graduate institution. Patients take the Goldman-Fristoe Test of Articulation 2 (Goldman & Fristoe, 2000) at baseline, and again after 16 weeks of treatment. Both the baseline and post-treatment standard scores are recorded. In addition, demographic information such as patient age at assessment, gender, and parents' education is obtained, along with at-home information such as average number of minutes the parents spent practicing with their child per day.

The data set is intended to be "realistic" in that it contains missing values for a variety of variables, as might occur in a typical data-collection scenario. Some patient records are missing noncritical variables, such as parents' education. In these cases, we examine a method of "filling in" these missing values where needed for estimation and predictive purposes. Other patients, however, may have dropped out of the clinic or moved away before the program was completed. These will have missing values for the post-treatment score, and may be removed before building regression models, for example.

One of the primary goals of this analysis is to explore whether and how the at-home practice time is associated with patient improvement in this particular sample, and to produce graphics for a report demonstrating the beneficial effect to parents and caregivers. An additional goal is to characterize the patient population in terms of relevant demographic factors and assess how these factors may be associated with patient outcome.

We now walk through a typical data analysis workflow in MATLAB, beginning with importing the clinical data as a `table` object. The data file itself is available for download from the textbook website, as is a script that contains all commands illustrated in the following sections.

Importing the Data

For simplicity, we assume the data file is uncreatively named "Clinical data.xlsx," and is stored under the "MATLAB" folder in the user's "Documents" folder or equivalent thereof (Figure 5–7).

As covered previously in this chapter, data can be imported to a `table` object by using the `readtable` function. In this case, the command would be

```
>> data = readtable('Clinical data.xlsx');
```

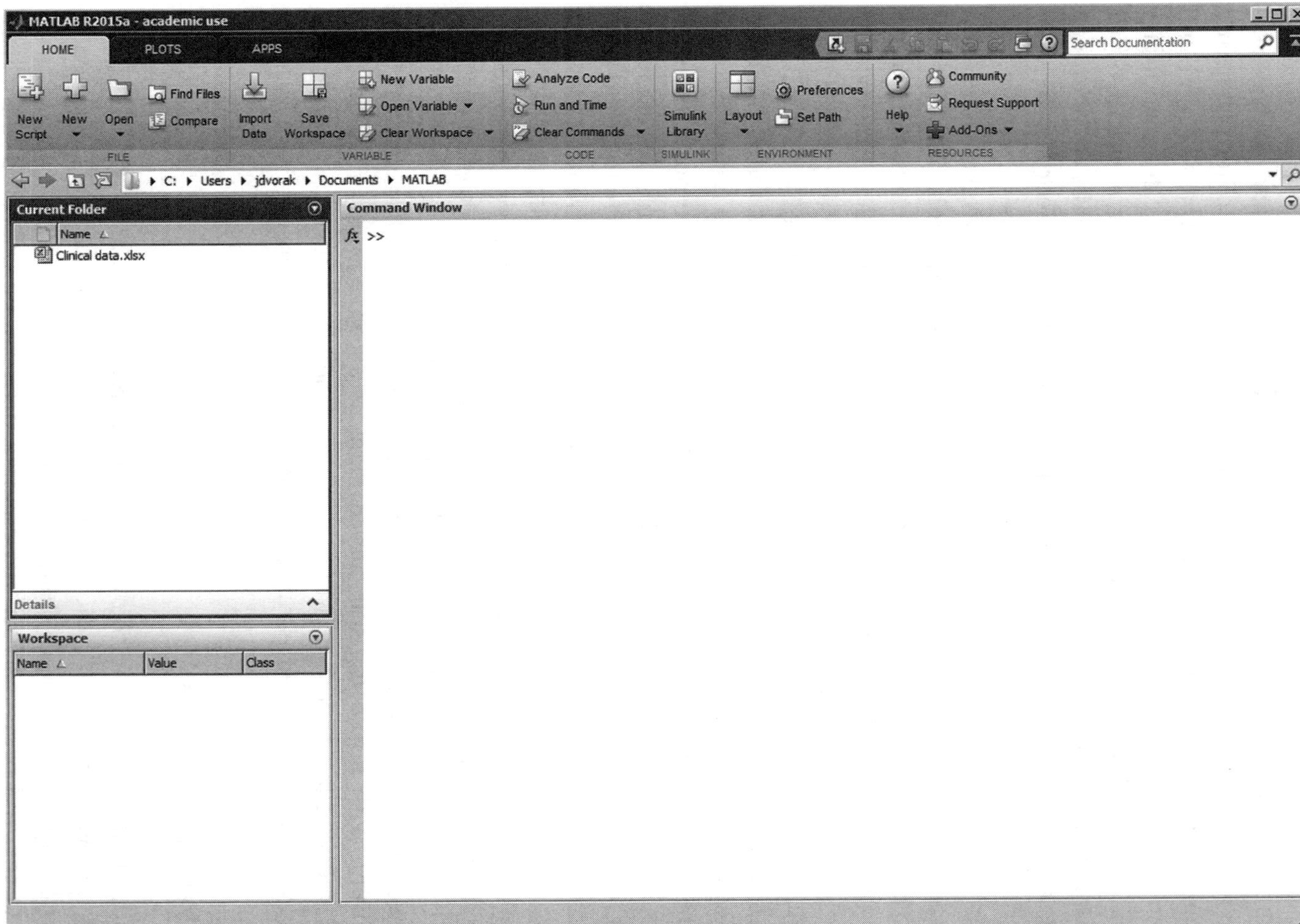

Figure 5–7. Expected setup for clinical scenario examples.

An alternative method of importing the data is simply dragging the Excel file into the Workspace and selecting the "Table" option under the "Import" tab when the "Import" window is displayed.

Exploring the Data

Now that the data set is imported, we can examine it using the `summary` function. Due to the number of variables, the output is not reproduced here, but it contains useful information as to the number of missing data points. In this example, there are three missing values for "parent/guardian 1 education," five missing values for "parent/guardian 2 education," and four missing post-treatment Goldman-Fristoe Test of Articulation 2 (GFTA-2; Goldman & Fristoe, 2000) scores, indicating four patients lost to follow-up.

Some demographic information can be extracted at this stage already. Suppose we are interested in the mean age of patients in years. The data set, as imported, has separate values for years and months, as is commonly recorded. To compute mean age, however, we need to determine a decimal value for years. This can be done by combining the two values as follows, overwriting the previous age in years:

```
>> data.AgeYears = data.AgeYears + data.AgeMonths/12;
```

At this point, we no longer need the months component, so we remove it from the data set using dot notation and an empty matrix (`[]`). By assigning an empty matrix to a variable in a `table` object, we can remove the column associated with that variable:

```
>> data.AgeMonths = [];
```

We now turn to the issue of the missing data points.

Imputation and Handling Missing Data

Imputation is the process of "filling" in blanks in a data set or table with reasonably selected values. A wide variety of imputation methods exist, as the field of imputation is relatively new and expanding. Although imputation theory is beyond the scope of this text, simple mean imputation can be performed in MATLAB and will be outlined in this section. In this method, missing values are replaced by the mean value or modal (i.e., most frequent) category in the data set, with optional stratification by relevant demographic groups or other grouping characteristics.

In our example data set, some demographic information is missing. This information is not only useful for describing the patient population, but may in fact be required for building predictive models of patient outcomes. This is because many modeling techniques such as, say, linear regression, require what is known as complete-case analysis. In complete-case analysis, only those cases (observations, patients, sessions, etc.) that are complete in all variables chosen as predictors will be used for modeling and subsequent prediction. Missing data for any variable in a case will exclude that case from analysis, thereby reducing the power of the statistical test performed. In our example, suppose we wish to use parents' education as a predictor in some model. Complete-case analysis would require ignoring 35% of our data set, which is inadvisable. Therefore, we seek some method to estimate or provide plausible values for the missing data.

In this example, we are interested in predicting the change in a patient's test score over a 16-week therapy program. For simplicity, we assume that any missing cells in the table are missing completely at random. This means that patients or parents from one group are no more or less likely to report their education status and demographic information and are also equally likely to be lost to follow-up (no post-treatment GFTA score). In this sample, all children are from two-parent households, so missing cells for parent/guardian education are taken to correspond to information that exists but was not provided. For flexibility, two slots in the data set are used for parent/guardian education regardless of gender or ordering.

To replace missing values with the sample mean, we must first identify the rows that do have missing values to begin with. This can be done with the `isnan` function, which returns `1` (indicating `true`) for missing data, and `0` (indicating `false`) for present data. The `nanmean` function, from the Statistics and Machine Learning Toolbox, computes the mean of a column or matrix of data after discarding missing values, which are coded internally in MATLAB as `NaN`. Combining the above, and using the results of `isnan` for logical indexing, the following commands perform mean imputation on both parents'/guardians' education level in years:

```
>> data.PG1Edu(isnan(data.PG1Edu)) = nanmean(data.PG1Edu);
>> data.PG2Edu(isnan(data.PG2Edu)) = nanmean(data.PG2Edu);
```

Although we might be tempted to impute values for the missing `PostGFTA` scores, doing so would be invalid. Here we must distinguish between "missing" data points, which arise from information that exists "out there" somewhere but was simply not recorded, and "empty" data points, which cannot ever be filled in because the corresponding values do not exist. In our scenario, there are no post-treatment scores since the patients were lost to follow-up. Therefore, we will likely need to remove these patients from the data set before performing complete-case modeling.

Removing or subsetting observations conditional on the value of a variable is a common operation, and it is worthwhile to spend some time examining it. Suppose we wish to remove all records corresponding to a patient with no post-treatment score. The `isnan` function is useful here, as it allows us to identify those rows which we want to exclude. By inverting its result with the negation operator ~, we acquire a column vector with ones for the observations to include, and zeros for those to exclude. Having done this, we then use the result to perform logical indexing of the `table` object. Just as with matrices, we use the : operator as the second element of the indexing expression to tell MATLAB to select all columns (variables):

```
>> goodRows = ~isnan(data.PostGFTA);
>> goodData = data(goodRows, :);
```

Subsetting is not only useful for excluding observations. It may be of use to perform an analysis after stratifying by a certain demographic factor. For example, suppose we wanted to examine males and females separately. A similar strategy applies: (a) construct a conditional expression that returns `1` for the rows we want to keep and `0` otherwise, (b) use logical indexing to select the rows from the master data set, and (c) assign the result to a new `table` object. Listing 5–4 illustrates the separation of the original data set into male and female subsets. Here we use the `strcmp` function because gender is stored as a series of strings.

Listing 5–4. Subsetting a data set

```
% Split into males vs. females.
malePts = strcmp(data.Gender, 'M');
femalePts = strcmp(data.Gender, 'F');
maleData = data(malePts, :);
femaleData = data(femalePts, :);
```

As an aside, if we are sure that gender is indicated for all patients, a more efficient way to extract the second data set would be to simply negate the logical indices used for the first one:

```
>> femalePts = data(~malePts, :);
```

Subsetting can be used to apply a more sophisticated method of imputation. If, for example, we had some suspicion that parents' educations were associated with some other demographic category (say, ZIP code or area code), we could perform subsetting on the data, do mean imputation within each subset, and then merge the data back using the `vertcat` function.

Simple Modeling and Testing

Having examined descriptive analysis of the data set, we now turn to the issue of modeling. Models can be used for two main purposes: (a) to test an a priori hypothesis about the data, or (b) to engage in pattern extraction and knowledge discovery.

In the first case, the entire data set (up to reasonable exclusions and imputations) is used to *support* or *reject* some predetermined hypothesis. It is important that the hypothesis be well-defined before any testing is conducted, lest one accidentally "confirm" a false-positive result due to noise in the data. For example, in our data set, we may wish to test the hypothesis that the average number of minutes per day of parental practice is associated with improvement over the course of the program. Note that this hypothesis would be generated by anecdotal clinical observations, and would not arise from the data set we are testing.

In the second case, it is common practice to split the data set into "training" and "testing" data sets. The training data set is used to detect patterns and associations, whereas the testing data set is used to check the model generated in the training set in an attempt to avoid overfitting. Overfitting occurs when the model "predicts" the data points within a given set with good accuracy, but fails to do so for a different set drawn from a similar population.

Example: Linear Regression

Linear regression models are used to detect and describe linear associations between continuous variables, such as measurements of age, test scores, and so on. In our example, we wish to determine whether a linear association exists between minutes of practice at home and improvement in scores relative to baseline. We first compute test improvement by forming the difference of the GFTA scores at baseline and post-treatment. Following mathematical tradition, we denote this as $\Delta GFTA$, or `DeltaGFTA` in MATLAB:

```
>> data.DeltaGFTA = data.PostGFTA - data.BaselineGFTA;
```

After performing this computation, a simple series of plotting commands (Listing 5–5) can display a scatterplot of the data (Figure 5–8). Note the usage

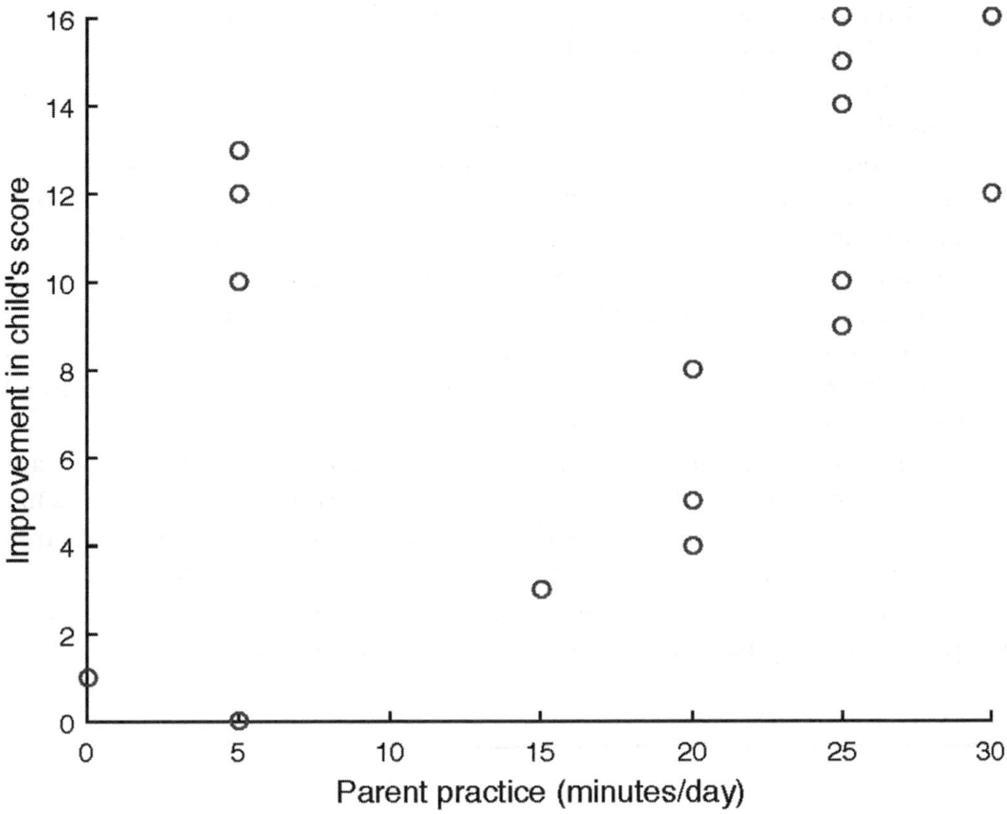

Figure 5–8. A scatter plot of clinical data.

of two apostrophes within the y-axis label string to avoid terminating the string early.

Listing 5–5. Plotting clinical data

```
scatter(data.MinutesPerDay, data.DeltaGFTA);
xlabel('Parent practice (minutes/day)');
ylabel('Improvement in child''s score');
```

We now use the `LinearModel.fit` function from the Statistics and Machine Learning Toolbox to fit a linear model. "Fitting" a model refers to the process of determining the optimum intercept and slope values for a line of the form $y = mx + b$, where y is the quantity we wish to predict and x is the variable we are using as a predictor. While a variety of methods exist for defining which combination is "optimal," the most common approach involves using the method of least squares, which attempts to minimize the squared vertical distance between the observed data points and the predicted values (i.e., the regression line) (Figure 5–9).

In this case, y denotes the change in GFTA score and x the average (reported) number of minutes spent practicing per day. The `LinearModel.fit` function requires us to specify the elements of the model using Wilkinson notation (Wilkinson & Rogers, 1973). The portion of this notation that will concern us involves specifying predicted versus predictor variables via the tilde character `'~'`. This is done by placing the predicted variable to the left of the tilde, the predictor(s) to the right, and enclosing the entire expression in single quotes to form a string. In this example, the model specification string is `'DeltaGFTA ~ MinutesPerDay'`. We tell MATLAB to fit a linear model of this form as shown in Figure 5–10.

After specifying the model and running the fitting algorithm, we are presented with a table of results. To the uninitiated, this can be somewhat intimidating; however, we are chiefly concerned in this case with only three pieces of information. The first is known as the p-value, which is an indicator of evidence in support of our original research question. A low p-value supports the proposed hypothesis, while a high p-value indicates lack of

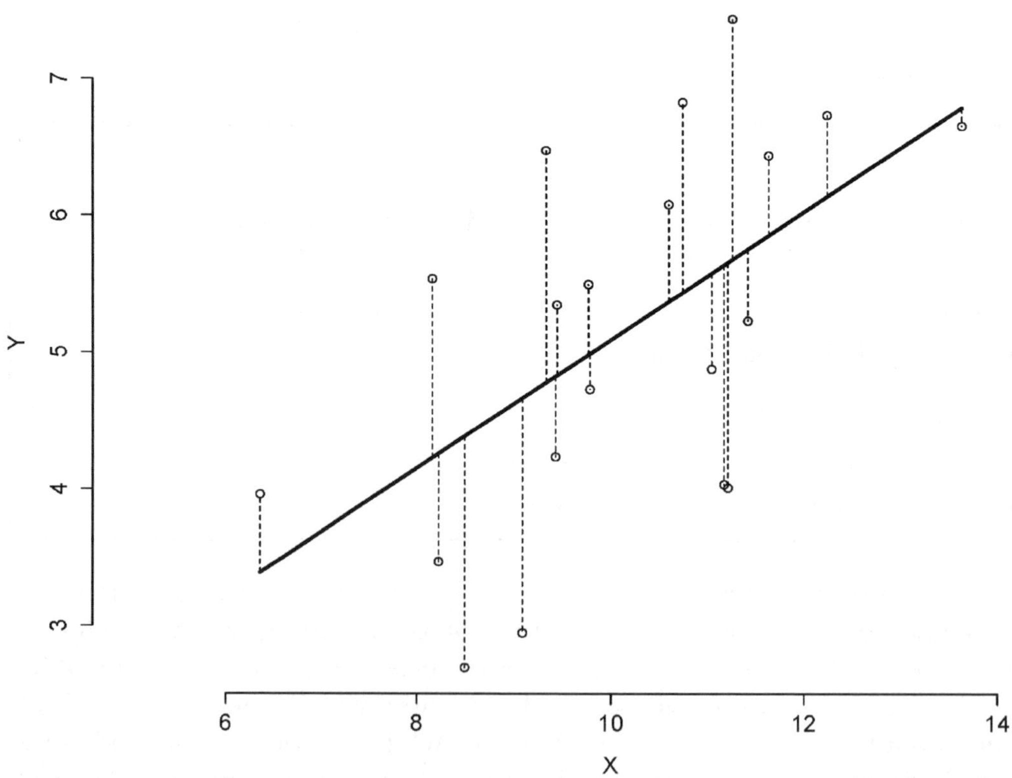

Figure 5–9. A regression line, as determined by least squares.

evidence for an effect. The *p*-value quantifies the probability that, assuming no true association exists, we would have observed results as or more extreme than the ones we have. It is traditional to consider results with a *p*-value of less than 0.05 to be "significant" (i.e., that they differ enough from what would be expected from chance). In this case, the association between minutes spent per day and test-score improvement is significant and positive, a point this hypothetical clinic's providers would do well to convey to administrators and parents.

The second quantity of interest is the R-squared value. This is the proportion of variation in the data that is explained by the linear relationship with the selected predictor. An R-squared of 1, while almost never seen in real data, suggests a perfect linear association. An R-squared of 0 indicates the lack of any linear association.

The final piece of information composes the coefficient estimates. These are the "best" values for m and b in the equation $y = mx + b$, and can be used to make predictions within the scope of the original data. In the example at hand, we would write

$$\hat{y} = 0.26x + 4.26$$

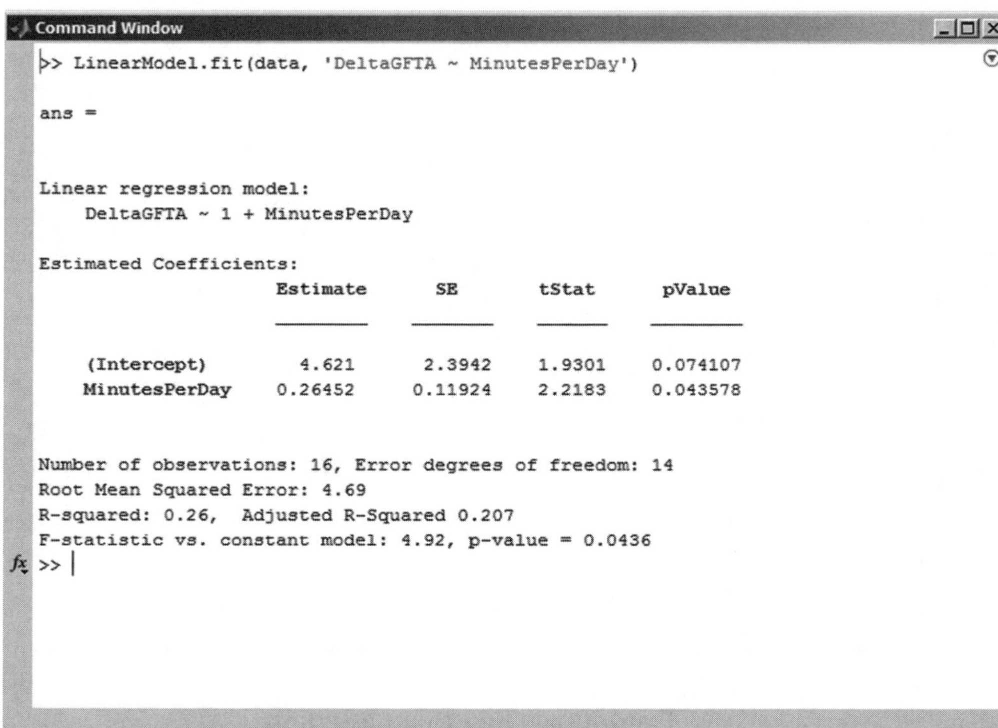

```
Command Window
>> LinearModel.fit(data, 'DeltaGFTA ~ MinutesPerDay')

ans =


Linear regression model:
    DeltaGFTA ~ 1 + MinutesPerDay

Estimated Coefficients:
                     Estimate     SE         tStat     pValue
                     ________     _______    ______    ________

    (Intercept)         4.621      2.3942    1.9301    0.074107
    MinutesPerDay     0.26452     0.11924    2.2183    0.043578


Number of observations: 16, Error degrees of freedom: 14
Root Mean Squared Error: 4.69
R-squared: 0.26,  Adjusted R-Squared 0.207
F-statistic vs. constant model: 4.92, p-value = 0.0436
>>
```

Figure 5–10. MATLAB output from linear regression modeling.

where the "hat" above y indicates that is a predicted value. To estimate a patient's overall improvement given his or her parents' reported minutes of practice per day, we would substitute minutes into x and compute $\hat{y}$.

Having fitted the model, we can be comfortable in superimposing the least-squares regression line specified therein (Figure 5–11). Figure 5–11 could be included in reports to clinic managers, or even shown to patients' parents/guardians to encourage sufficient practice. A least-squares line can be easily superimposed on an existing scatterplot through the use of the `lsline` function from the Statistics and Machine Learning Toolbox:

```
>> lsline();
```

Although of great importance to data mining, the topics of multiple linear regression, checking model assumptions, and statistical inference in general are beyond the scope of this text; readers are advised to consult statistical textbooks (e.g., Kutner, Nachtsheim, Neter, & Li, 2004) for more information before attempting to fit complex models.

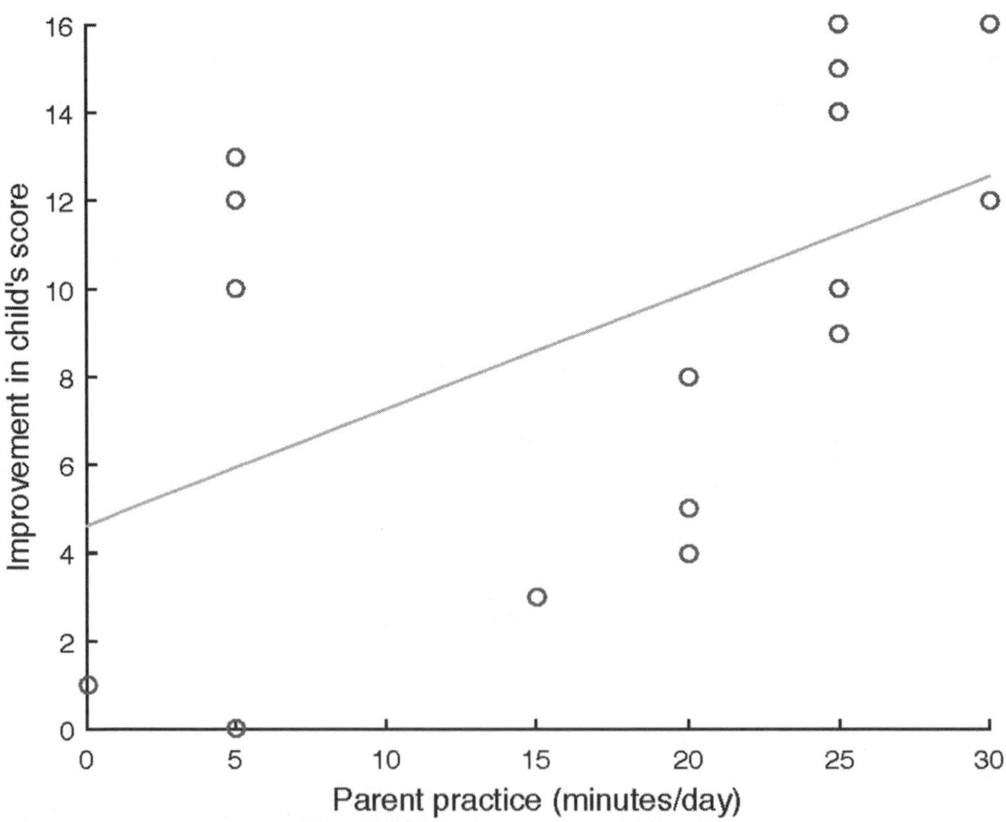

Figure 5–11. Superimposing a least-squares regression line.

Example: *k*-Means Clustering

Clustering involves grouping records from a data set so that records within a cluster are more similar to one another than to records in another cluster, where the operational definition of "similar" varies by the algorithm chosen. It can be used, for example, to identify important patient subgroups within a clinic's target population, or even to discover the appropriate number of groups that one should use, given the data at hand. By understanding the demographic and clinical "behavior" of patient clusters, clinicians and supervisors can be better equipped to make more informed judgements.

As a machine-learning algorithm, clustering is data driven rather than hypothesis driven. That is, one begins with a data set and uses clustering to discover patterns. If we do not already know the clusters or categories to begin with (i.e., we are trying to discover them from the data), then the process of generating the clusters falls under the broader category of unsupervised machine learning. This contrasts with statistical classification, in which the "correct" category is known and we are more interested in predicting a result for a new patient.

A variety of clustering algorithms are used in data mining, the appropriate selection of which is often left to the investigator's judgement based on the task at hand (Estivill-Castro, 2002). For this exercise, we focus on *k*-means clustering, which is classified as a centroid-based clustering model.

k-means clustering involves the separation of data points into a predefined number *k* of clusters (Bramer, 2013). Separation requires the generation of cluster centroids, which are ideal "members" of the data set that lie at the center of the cluster. Points are then assigned to a cluster if they are closer to its centroid than they are to any other cluster's centroid. In this sense, "closer" is usually defined as the *d*-dimensional Euclidean distance between the point and the proposed centroid, where *d* indicates the number of variables on which the clustering is performed (i.e., the dimensionality). As a speech example, one might wish to cluster patients by age and standardized baseline GFTA scores to discover trends in a patient population.

In audiology, Anwar, Oakes, Wermter, and Heinrich (2010) have applied *k*-means clustering to audiogram data to determine which patients would benefit most from receiving a hearing aid, and compute the ideal number of clusters to use by means of the silhouette method, a technique that will be explored shortly.

After selecting *k*, the next step is to define a way to measure how "good" the clustering is. This is done through specification of an **objective function**. For optimization problems in general, the objective function measures the distance of the proposed solution from the optimal or best case. The output of the function is used for the purposes of minimizing this distance. In *k*-means clustering, a common objective function to use is the sum of squared distances between each point and its cluster's centroid (Bramer, 2013). In the ideal case, for example, all points within a cluster would be located at the same position in the *d*-dimensional space, giving a distance of 0. In real applications, this is quite rare, but minimizing this distance can aid an algorithm in deciding on the best position for the centroids.

With *k* and the objective function defined, *k*-means algorithms then begin by randomly selecting *k* points and setting these as the centroids of the clusters. Each remaining point is then assigned to the same cluster as the centroid closest to it. After all points are assigned to clusters, the centroids for each cluster are recomputed, and the process is repeated until there is no change in the centroids.

While the initial centroids and clusters are quite unlikely to be ideal, the iterative process refines the results until they can no longer improve relative to their current position. This "relative" improvement is important, as the initial setting of centroids can result in different clusters. Therefore, it is common to perform several runs of *k*-means clustering for each value of *k*, with the best clusters being selected as those whose final form minimizes the objective function.

In MATLAB, *k*-means clustering can be performed easily with the `kmeans` function from the Statistics and Machine Learning Toolbox. As a technical note, this function uses a more efficient means of selecting the initial centroids than the random approach discussed above; this updated approach is known as the *k*-means++ algorithm (Arthur & Vassilvitskii, 2007).

Suppose we wish to cluster patients based on our previous variables of interest (improvement on the GFTA and number of minutes spent on practice per night), and that we are interested in seeing how well a *k* of 2 describes the data (Listing 5–6). This is accomplished as follows (assume that the table `data` has been cleaned of missing observations), with the caveat that the `kmeans` function requires a matrix of data, which we assemble here by using dot notation and combining the two column vectors `data.MinutesPerDay` and `data.DeltaGFTA` into a single matrix. Note that $k = 2$ has nothing to do with the fact that we selected two variables; we could have selected 3, 4, or even dozens of variables while leaving *k* at 2.

Listing 5–6. Application of *k*-means clustering to clinical data

```
% Do k-means clustering for k=2.
[clusterNum, centroids] = kmeans([data.MinutesPerDay, data.DeltaGFTA], 2);

% Plot clusters.
plot(data.MinutesPerDay(clusterNum==1), ...
    data.DeltaGFTA(clusterNum==1), 'b+');
hold on;
```

```
scatter(data.MinutesPerDay(clusterNum==2), ...
    data.DeltaGFTA(clusterNum==2), 'ro');
xlabel('Average daily practice (minutes)')
ylabel('Change in GFTA from baseline')

% Plot centroids.
plot(centroids(1, 1), centroids(1, 2), ...
    'b+', 'MarkerSize', 10, 'LineWidth', 3)
plot(centroids(2, 1), centroids(2, 2), ...
    'ro', 'MarkerSize', 10, 'LineWidth', 3)
```

The results of this clustering are displayed in Figure 5–12, with each data point's cluster membership indicated by the use of a different symbol. Centroids for a given cluster are indicated by larger versions of the corresponding symbol.

However, this still leaves open the question of whether two is the ideal number of clusters for this data set. For example, perhaps a valid reason exists

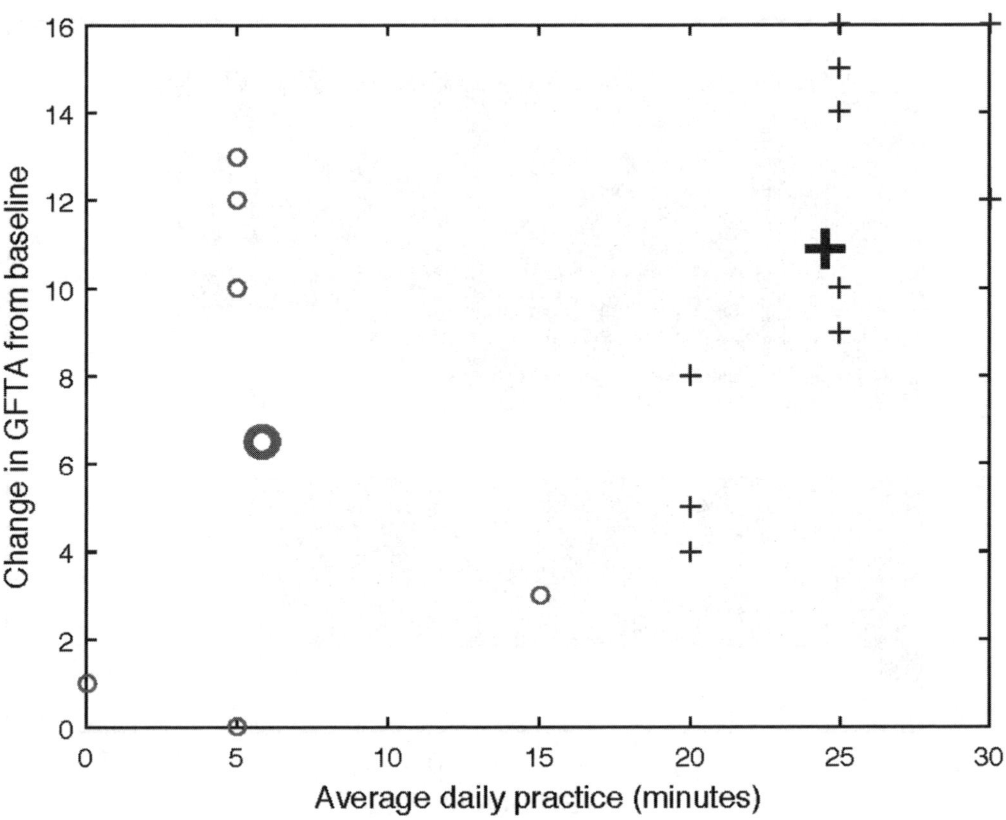

Figure 5–12. Clustering results.

for the selection of three or even more clusters. One naïve approach might be to use the original objective function and see which number of clusters minimizes it. However, moderate consideration leads to the conclusion that, as the number of clusters approaches the number of data points, the objective function will approach zero. In fact, if $k = n$, all points are exactly at the centroid of their "clusters," so the objective function is exactly zero. This is analogous to overfitting as discussed previously, in that it provides a "good" result for exactly the data at hand, but does not generalize to new observations or patient populations.

A large variety of indices have been developed for the purpose of selecting the number of clusters for cluster analysis (see, for example, Dimitriadou, Dolnicar, & Weingessel, 2002). One such index is based on a graphical tool known as the silhouette plot, which can be produced with the MATLAB function `silhouette` after performing initial clustering. The silhouette plot for the two-cluster scenario above (Figure 5–13) is produced as follows:

```
>> silhouette([data.MinutesPerDay, data.DeltaGFTA], clusterNum);
```

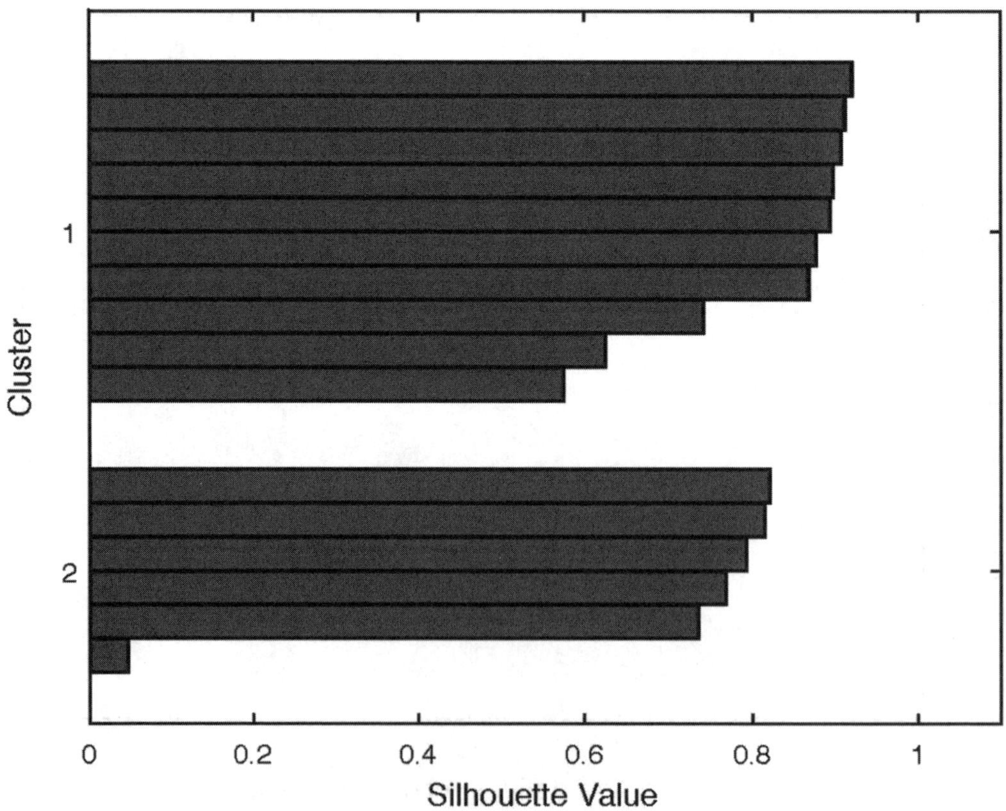

Figure 5–13. A silhouette plot.

Interpreting this plot involves looking for silhouette values near 1, meaning that the points are close to their centroids and far from the cluster boundary. A silhouette value of zero means the opposite, namely, that the point is close to the boundary and therefore questionably clustered. A quantitative way to measure the quality of clustering via silhouette plots is to compute the mean silhouette values.

As with many other operations in MATLAB, this computation can be automated for the purposes of determining an outcome, in this case the "best" number of clusters. Note that the value selected from this process is not necessarily the best for all possible cases or clinical scenarios, and in fact can be quite far from the truth. One should always visually inspect the clusters, as well as apply domain knowledge for a sanity test, before blindly relying on an algorithm. That being said, Listing 5–7 is an efficient way to pick out a suggestion for the ideal number of clusters.

Listing 5–7. Automation of silhouette value computation for selecting *k*

```
% Try to detect ideal number of clusters.
ks = 2:6;
silMeans = zeros(length(ks), 1);
for i = 1:length(ks)
    % Perform k-means clustering.
    k = ks(i);
    [clusterNum, centroids] = kmeans([data.MinutesPerDay, ...
        data.DeltaGFTA], k);

    % Note: One should plot the clusters and centroids for visual
    % inspection, but that code (see previous listing) is removed for
    % brevity.

    % Determine silhouette values.
    s = silhouette([data.MinutesPerDay, data.DeltaGFTA], clusterNum);

    % Compute average silhouette score.
    silMeans(i) = mean(s);

end

% Plot mean silhouette score by k.
plot(ks, silMeans)
xlabel('k')
ylabel('Mean silhouette score')
```

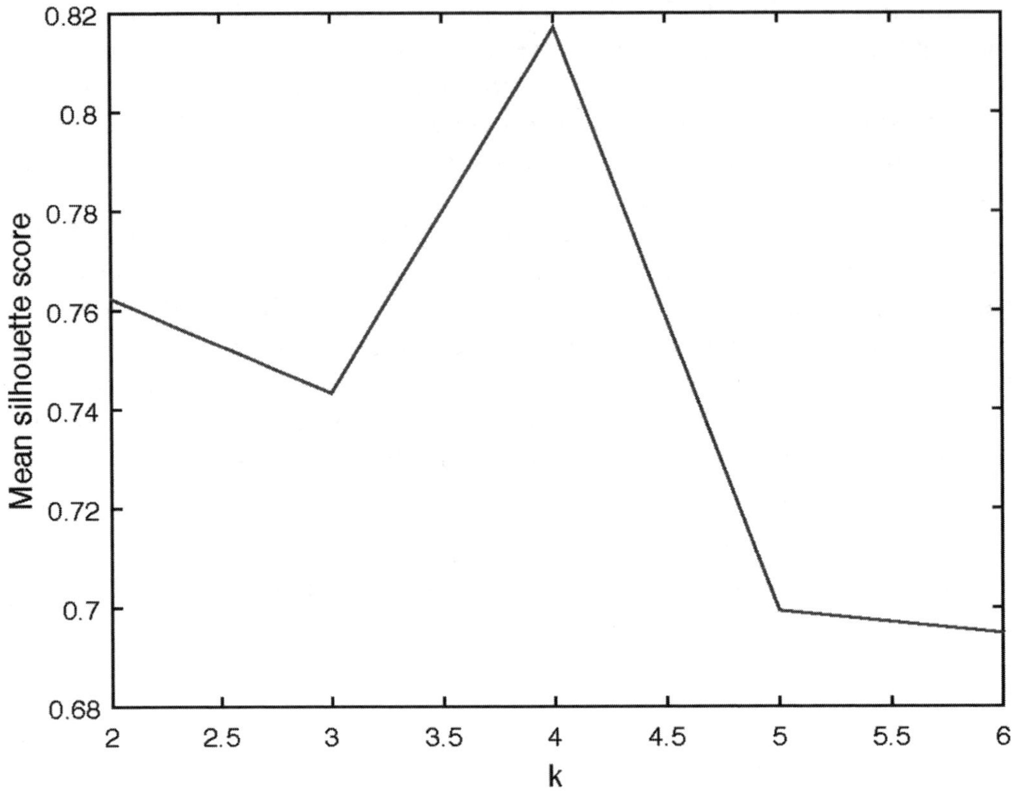

Figure 5–14. Automated selection of *k* by silhouette values.

For this data set, the average silhouette value plot (Figure 5–14) suggests a *k* of 4. Again, caution is advised in blindly accepting this number due to the small sample size used (clustering often involves hundreds or thousands of observations).

References

Anwar, N., Oakes, M., Wermter, S., & Heinrich, S. (2010). *Clustering audiology data.* Paper presented at the 19th Annual Machine Learning Conference of Belgium and The Netherlands, Leuven, NL.

Arthur, D., & Vassilvitskii, S. (2007). K-means++: The advantages of careful seeding. In *Proceedings of the Eighteenth Annual ACM-SIAM Symposium on Discrete Algorithms,* 2007 (pp. 1027–1035). Philadelphia, PA: Society for Industrial and Applied Mathematics.

Bramer, M. (2013). *Principles of data mining* (2nd ed.). New York, NY: Springer.

Broughton, W., Lashlee, H., Marcum, C., & Mustata-Wilson, G. (2013). Health information technology: A new world of nursing homes. *Journal of Gerontology & Geriatric Research, 2*, 122.

Cebul, R. D., Love, T. E., Jain, A. K., & Hebert, C. J. (2011). Electronic health records and quality of diabetes care. *New England Journal of Medicine, 365*(9), 825–833.

Cleophas, T. J., & Zwinderman, A. H. (2015). *Machine learning in medicine—A complete overview*. New York, NY: Springer.

Congressional Budget Office (CBO). (2008, May). *Evidence on the costs and benefits of health information technology*. Washington, DC: CBO.

Dimitriadou, E., Dolnicar, S., & Weingessel, A. (2002). An examination of indexes for determining the number of clusters in binary data sets. *Psychometrica, 67*(3), 137–160.

Estivill-Castro, V. (2002). Why so many clustering algorithms—A position paper. *ACM SIGKDD Explorations Newsletter, 4*(1), 65–75.

Fayyad, U., Piatetsky-Shapiro, G., & Smyth, P. (1996). From data mining to knowledge discovery in databases. *AI Magazine, 17*(3), 37–54.

Frawley, W. J., Piatetsky-Shapiro, G., & Matheus, C. J. (1992). Knowledge discovery in databases: An overview. *AI Magazine, 13*(3), 57–70.

Goldman, R., & Fristoe, M. (2000). *Goldman-Fristoe Test of Articulation 2*. San Antonio, TX: Pearson.

Gunter, T. D., & Terry, N. P. (2005). The emergence of national electronic health records in the United States and Australia: Models, costs, and questions. *Journal of Medical Internet Research, 7*(1), e3.

Himmelstein, D. U., Wright, A., & Woolhandler, S. (2010). Hospital computing and the costs and quality of care: A national study. *American Journal of Medicine, 123*(1), 40–46.

Kutner, M., Nachtsheim, C., Neter, J., & Li, W. (2004). *Applied linear statistical models* (5th ed.). Columbus, OH: McGraw-Hill.

Liu, D., & Nicholas, G. C. (2009). Health information technology in nursing homes. *Journal of Applied Gerontology, 28*, 38–58.

Wilkinson, G. N., & Rogers, C. E. (1973). Symbolic description of factorial models for analysis of variance. *Journal of the Royal Statistical Society, Series C (Applied Statistics), 22*(3), 392–399.

APPENDIX A

Review of Trigonometry

Several trigonometric concepts are essential for understanding the fundamentals of signal processing and simple harmonic motion. Among these are sine waves, radians, and angular frequency. This section does not attempt a complete review of trigonometry, but it instead aims to present these key concepts to further the reader's understanding of the main text.

Trigonometry is often discussed in terms of the "unit circle," which is a circle of radius 1 centered at the origin of a Cartesian (i.e., *X-Y*) plane. For the purposes of computation of trigonometric functions, angles are commonly measured in radians from the positive *x*-axis in a counterclockwise direction. Starting from the relation $c = 2\pi r$, where c is the circumference of a circle and r is its radius, we have $c = 2\pi$ for the unit circle. An angle's measure in radians, then, is simply the arc length it subtends on the circle. An angle θ in radians can be computed from an angle a in degrees as follows:

$$\theta = \frac{2\pi}{360^\circ}a = \frac{\pi}{180^\circ}a$$

In Figure A–1 is depicted a unit circle with an angle subtending 45 degrees, or $\pi/4$ radians.

The dashed line represents the positive *x*-axis, whereas the solid line represents the hypotenuse of a right triangle whose 45° angle is located at the origin. The dotted line marked "x" is the horizontal component. The dotted line marked "y" is the vertical component.

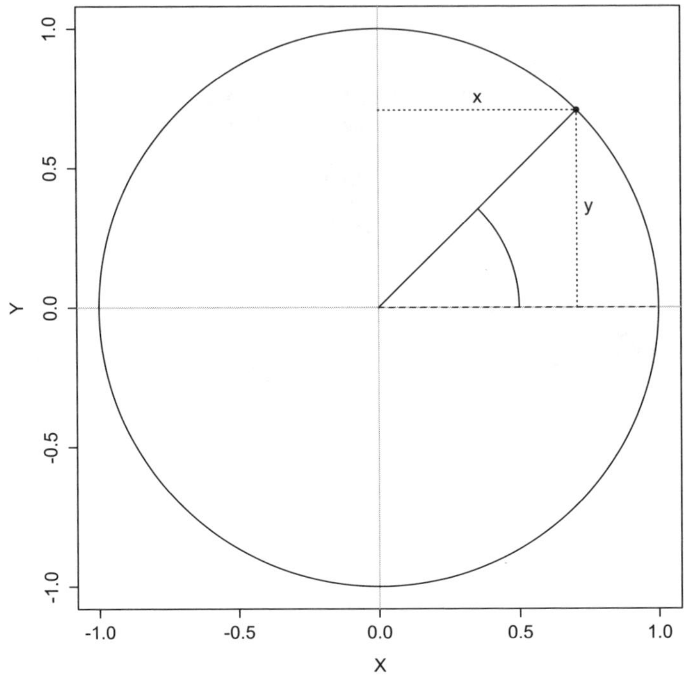

Figure A–1. Unit circle.

Suppose we have a particle moving counterclockwise along the circle. This particle moves in such a way that the angle to it increases by a constant rate, denoted ω. For a particle completing one revolution per second, we have $\omega = 2\pi$, because in one second the particle will have traversed the complete circumference of the circle. Just as degrees can be converted to radians, so too can a frequency f in cps or Hz be converted to an angular frequency ω:

$$\omega = 2\pi f$$

If we plot the vertical component of such a particle in terms of time, we have a sine wave. In Figure A–2, the *x*-axis represents time in seconds, and the *y*-axis the particle's current vertical displacement from zero. Since $\omega = 2\pi$, we have $f = 1$, yielding a simple 1-Hz sine wave.

Mathematically, Figure A–2 can be represented as $y = \sin(2\pi t)$, where t is the time in seconds. For any sine wave with frequency f and corresponding angular frequency ω, we have

$$y = \sin(2\pi ft) = \sin(\omega t)$$

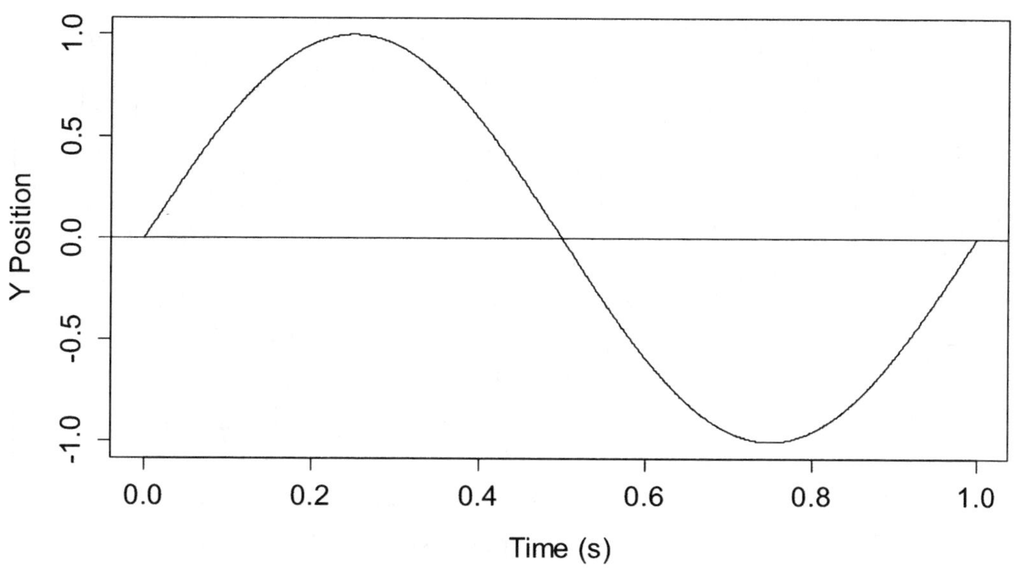

Figure A–2. Sine wave.

The period of a sine wave, denoted T, is the inverse of its frequency. Note that care must be taken when dealing with units other than seconds. In this case, we have a period of 1 second, or 1000 milliseconds:

$$T = \frac{1}{f} = \frac{1}{1\text{ Hz}} = \frac{1}{1\left(\frac{\text{cycle}}{\text{s}}\right)} = 1\frac{\text{s}}{\text{cycle}} = 1$$

For the sine wave in Figure A–3, the computation of the period is less straightforward. Let $f = 15$ Hz.

In this case, $T = \frac{1}{15} = 0.0667$ s = 66.7 ms.

When discussing the frequencies and waveforms of interest for human speech, it is often more convenient to represent period in terms of milliseconds than seconds. For example, taking an average male vocal tract of 17.5 cm with an approximant first formant frequency of 500 Hz, we have $T = \frac{1}{500} = 0.002$ s = 2 ms, which denotes the time required for the necessary propagation of compression and rarefaction waves within the vocal tract to produce one complete cycle.

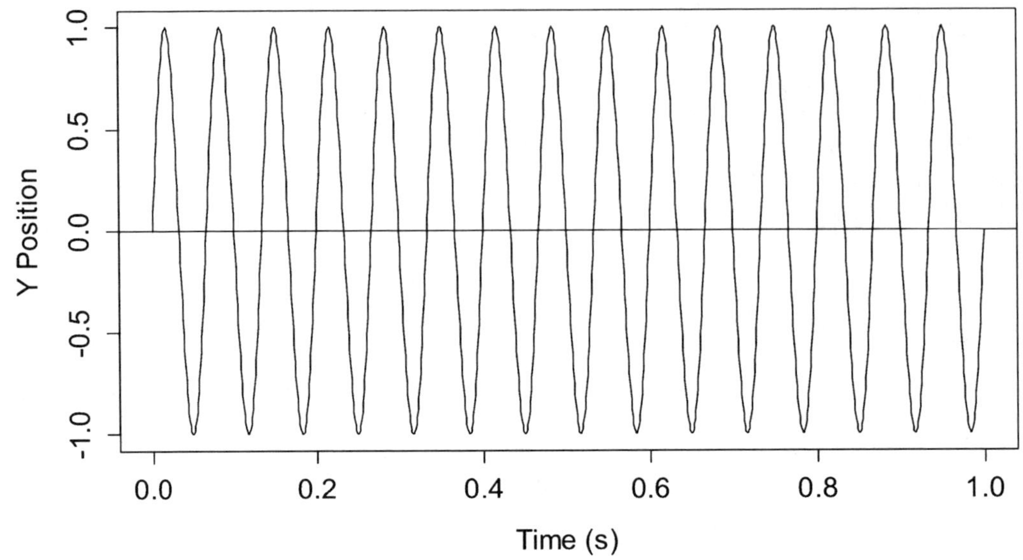

Figure A–3. Sine wave.

APPENDIX B

Review of Complex Numbers

The mathematical foundation behind the analysis of signals, Fourier transforms, results in a set of complex-valued coefficients. As such, an understanding of complex numbers is beneficial in using this technique. This appendix presents a brief review of key concepts in the use and manipulation of complex numbers.

Complex numbers are those with a *real* and an *imaginary* component. The real component of a complex number is what non-mathematicians may call a "normal," "regular," or "decimal" number, and it can be represented as a point on the number line or *real line*, whether negative or positive (Figure B–1).

The imaginary unit, denoted i or j, is defined as the solution to the equation $i^2 = -1$. Such solutions arose in the manipulation of polynomials, and philosophers such as Descartes (1637) used the term "imaginary" to contrast these numbers to the more concrete real numbers. Despite the name, imaginary numbers are quite "real" in a mathematical and algorithmic sense, and provide a critical abstraction allowing the solution of important equations.

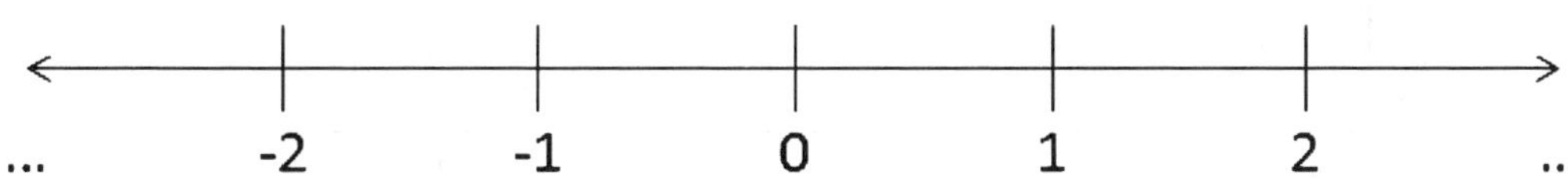

Figure B–1. The real line.

In particular, Euler's formula relates complex numbers and trigonometric functions, stating that

$$e^{i\theta} = \cos(\theta) + i\sin(\theta)$$

Complex numbers, of the form $z = a + bi$, are not plotted on the number line alone; rather, they are plotted on the complex plane. Traditionally, the horizontal axis denotes the real component Re(z), and the vertical axis denotes the imaginary component, denoted Im(z) (Figure B–2).

One important equation in speech analysis concerns the relationship between time and frequency in the analysis of sampled speech signals, and it is known as the discrete Fourier transform. Below is reproduced the defining equation for this transform, where y denotes the original speech signal sample at time n, N denotes the total number of samples in the signal, Y_k denotes the complex value of the transform for a given integer k in the interval $[0, N-1]$, and i denotes the complex unit described above. A popular convention in MATLAB programming uses capitalized versions of the variable name to represent discrete Fourier transform (DFT) transformations of the original signal:

$$Y_k = \sum_{n=0}^{N} \left[y_n e^{\frac{-2\pi ikn}{N}} \right]$$

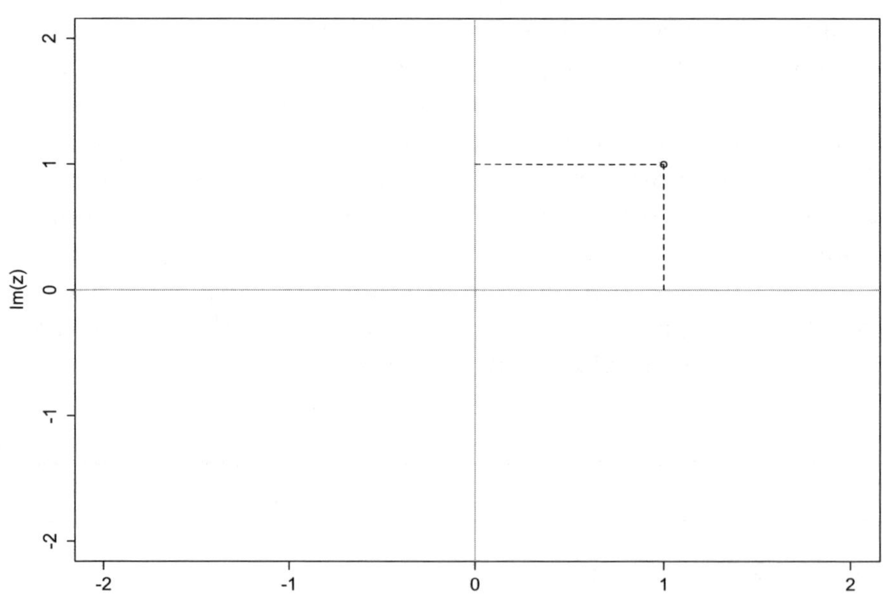

Figure B–2. Complex plot of $z = 1 + 1i$.

By Euler's identity, it can be seen that the discrete Fourier transform results in a set of real and imaginary sine and cosine components:

$$Y_k = \sum_{n=0}^{N} \left[y_n e^{i\left(\frac{-2\pi kn}{N}\right)} \right] = \sum_{n=0}^{N} \left[y_n \cos\left(\frac{-2\pi kn}{N}\right) + y_n i \sin\left(\frac{-2\pi kn}{N}\right) \right]$$

Each element of the transformed vector Y is a complex number, having a real and imaginary component, and represents both the amplitude and phase of the selected frequency, averaged across the entire signal. The *amplitude* of a given frequency element (also termed the *modulus*, although this is not to be confused with modular arithmetic) is computed as

$$r = |Y_k| = \sqrt{a_k^2 + b_k^2}$$

The *phase* (also termed *argument*) of a given frequency element is found by determining the angle subtended by a line drawn from the origin of the complex plane to the point in question, and is the solution to the system of equations:

$$r_k \sin(\phi_k) = b_k$$

$$r_k \cos(\phi_k) = a_k$$

MATLAB allows easy computation of the fast Fourier transform (FFT) of a signal through the use of the `fft()` function, and extraction of amplitude and phase through `abs()` and `arg()`. Note that in analyzing human speech, relative phase information is often of little importance for recognition and is generally ignored in computing spectra and spectrograms.

APPENDIX C

Review of Matrices

Matrices lie at the heart of MATLAB and are useful abstractions for storing arrangements of numeric data. Of particular importance to speech-language pathologists wishing to analyze speech are matrices stored as .wav files. These matrices often have two columns (one for each channel) and thousands of rows. Efficient programming in terms of matrices is facilitated by an understanding of some of the key mathematical principles underlying them. As such, these principles are summarized here.

For the purposes of speech analysis, a matrix is simply a two-dimensional array or grid of numbers. Matrices are often denoted as

$$M = \begin{bmatrix} a & b \\ c & d \\ \vdots & \vdots \end{bmatrix}$$

where *a*, *b*, and so on are termed *elements* of the matrix *M*. Single numbers are termed *scalars* in contrast with matrices. An element's location within a matrix is described by its row and column, starting with 1:

		Column 1	Column 2
Row	1	*a*	*b*
	2	*c*	*d*
	⋮	⋮	⋮

In the example above, a is in the cell $M_{1,1}$ and b is in the cell $M_{1,2}$. MATLAB uses this same style of row/column indexing to allow users to access elements in a specific position:

```
>> M = [1, 2, 3; 4, 5, 6]

M =

     1     2     3
     4     5     6

>> M(2, 1)

ans =

     4

>> M(2, 3) = 7 % Assigns 7 to cell (2, 3) in M.

M =

     1     2     3
     4     5     7
```

Common operations on matrices include addition, subtraction, multiplication, division, and transposition.

Addition and subtraction can be performed only for matrices matching in both dimensions. In such cases, the operation is performed element-wise:

$$\begin{bmatrix} 1 & 3 \\ 2 & 4 \end{bmatrix} + \begin{bmatrix} 2 & 4 \\ 6 & 8 \end{bmatrix} = \begin{bmatrix} 1+2 & 3+4 \\ 2+6 & 4+8 \end{bmatrix} = \begin{bmatrix} 3 & 7 \\ 8 & 12 \end{bmatrix}$$

As with scalars, addition is commutative. That is, the order of matrices does not matter. Subtraction, however, is not commutative.

Multiplication for matrices is somewhat more complicated than addition. When a scalar is multiplied by a matrix, as in $N = aM$, the scalar multiple is applied element-wise:

$$a = 5$$

$$M = \begin{bmatrix} 1 & 3 \\ 2 & 4 \end{bmatrix}$$

$$N = aM = 5\begin{bmatrix} 1 & 3 \\ 2 & 4 \end{bmatrix} = \begin{bmatrix} 5 & 15 \\ 10 & 20 \end{bmatrix}$$

When two matrices are multiplied, the result (and even its existence) depends on which definition of multiplication is being used. The easiest type of matrix multiplication to compute, although not necessarily the most commonly applied, is known as the Hadamard product or Schur product. This is the multiplicative analogue to the element-wise addition described above, and is denoted $M \circ N$ for two matrices of the same dimensions. For example,

$$M = \begin{bmatrix} 0 & 1 \\ 2 & 3 \end{bmatrix}$$

$$N = \begin{bmatrix} 1 & 2 \\ 3 & 4 \end{bmatrix}$$

$$M \circ N = \begin{bmatrix} 0 \times 1 & 1 \times 2 \\ 2 \times 3 & 3 \times 4 \end{bmatrix} = \begin{bmatrix} 0 & 2 \\ 6 & 12 \end{bmatrix}$$

The Hadamard product can be applied in MATLAB with the `.*` symbol as follows:

```
>> M = [0, 1; 2, 3]

M =

     0     1
     2     3

>> N = [1, 2; 3, 4]

N =

     1     2
     3     4

>> M .* N

ans =

     0     2
     6    12
```

This operation is mainly useful when vectorizing code to perform many permutations of products. For example, suppose we want to create a sum of sinewaves to synthesize sinewave speech, and need to multiply each frequency component by a particular amplitude to achieve the correct formant structure. This can be done as follows (Listing C–1):

Listing C–1. Synthesis of sinewaves

```
% Define formant values.
formants = [500, 1500, 2500];
numFormants = length(formants);

% Define amplitudes.
amps = [0.5, 0.25, 0.125];

% Create a one-second "vowel" at 1000 samples/sec.
numSamples = 1000;
time = linspace(0, 1, numSamples)';

% Repeat the times vector by the number of formants.
times = repmat(time, 1, numFormants);

% Repeat the frequencies vector by the length of time.
freqs = repmat(formants, numSamples, 1);

% Repeat the amplitude vector.
amps = repmat(amps, numSamples, 1);

% Generate the scaled sine waves using elementwise multiplication.
y = amps .* sin(2 * pi * freqs .* times);
```

The most common definition of matrix multiplication, however, is termed the *matrix product* and is denoted simply as *MN*. If two matrices are to be multiplied in this fashion, their inner dimensions must match. This means that the number of columns of the first matrix must be equal to the number of rows in the second. Unlike with scalars, matrix multiplication is not necessarily commutative, and may not be defined for all combinations of matrices.

The matrix product in MATLAB is found with the * symbol:

```
>> M = [0, 1; 2, 3]

M =

     0     1
     2     3
```

```
>> N = [1, 2; 3, 4]

N =

     1     2
     3     4

>> M * N

ans =

     3     4
    11    16
```

Matrix transposition involves the interchanging of rows and columns. This can often be a useful technique when plotting data, as MATLAB will automatically plot a matrix column-wise. Two notations exist to indicate a transposed matrix:

$$M = \begin{bmatrix} 1 & 4 & 9 \\ 16 & 25 & 36 \end{bmatrix}$$

$$M^T = M' = \begin{bmatrix} 1 & 16 \\ 4 & 25 \\ 9 & 36 \end{bmatrix}$$

In MATLAB, these notations are reflected with two commands, which are equivalent in the case of real numbers:

```
>> M = [1, 4, 9; 16, 25, 36]

M =

     1     4     9
    16    25    36

>> M'

ans =

     1    16
     4    25
     9    36
```

```
>> transpose(M)

ans =

     1    16
     4    25
     9    36
```

APPENDIX D

Source Code for an Interactive Spectral-Analysis GUI

```
function spectralGUI()

    f = figure('Name', 'Simple spectral analysis GUI', ...
        'Units', 'Norm', ...
        'NumberTitle', 'off', ...
        'MenuBar', 'None', ...
        'ToolBar', 'Figure');

    % Set up UI controls.
    startButton = uicontrol(f, 'Style', 'PushButton', ...
        'String', 'Start recording', ...
        'Units', 'Norm', ...
        'Position', [0, 0, 1/3, 0.125], ...
        'Callback', @startRecording);
    stopButton = uicontrol(f, 'Style', 'PushButton', ...
        'String', 'Stop recording', ...
        'Units', 'Norm', ...
        'Position', [1/3, 0, 1/3, 0.125], ...
        'Callback', @stopRecording, ...
```

```
    'Enable', 'off');
playButton = uicontrol(f, 'Style', 'PushButton', ...
    'String', 'Play recorded sample', ...
    'Units', 'Norm', ...
    'Position', [2/3, 0, 1/3, 1/8], ...
    'Callback', @playSample, ...
    'Enable', 'off');

% Set up menus.
m = uimenu(f, 'Label', 'File');
hOpen = uimenu(m, 'Label', 'Open...', ...
    'Callback', @openFile);
hSave = uimenu(m, 'Label', 'Save as...', ...
    'Callback', @saveFile);
hExport = uimenu(m, 'Label', 'Export to workspace', ...
    'Callback', @toWorkspace);

% Set up placeholders for speech and spectral data.
fs = 44100;
time = (1:fs) / fs * 1000;
y = zeros(1, fs);
NFFT = 2^nextpow2(fs);
freqs = fs/2 * linspace(0, 1, NFFT/2 + 1) / 1000;
amps = zeros(1, length(freqs));
freqsLow = freqs(freqs <= 1) * 1000;
ampsLow = amps(freqs <= 1);

% Set up waveform plot.
hWave = axes('Parent', f, 'OuterPosition', [0, 10/16, 0.5, 6/16]);
pWave = plot(hWave, time, y);
ylim(hWave, [-1, 1])
title(hWave, 'Waveform plot')
xlabel(hWave, 'Time (ms)')
ylabel(hWave, 'Y')

% Set up spectrogram plot.
fsSG = 10000;
hSG = axes('Parent', f, 'OuterPosition', [0, 3/16, 0.5, 7/16]);
WINDOW = floor(fsSG/10);
NOVERLAP = ceil(fsSG/20);
NFFTSG = 2^nextpow2(WINDOW);
[S, F, T] = spectrogram(y, WINDOW, NOVERLAP, NFFTSG, fsSG, 'yaxis');
```

```
S = zeros(length(F), length(T));
hIm = image(T*1000, F/1000, S, 'Parent', hSG);
set(hIm, 'CDataMapping', 'scaled')
axis(hSG, 'xy');
%colormap(hSG, flipud(gray));
xlabel(hSG, 'Time (ms)')
ylabel(hSG, 'Frequency (kHz)')
title(hSG, 'Spectrogram')

% Set up spectrum plot.
hSpect = axes('Parent', f, 'OuterPosition', [0.5, 10/16, 0.5, 6/16]);
pSpect = plot(hSpect, freqs, amps);
ylim(hSpect, [0, 1])
title(hSpect, 'Amplitude spectrum')
xlabel(hSpect, 'Frequency (kHz)')
ylabel(hSpect, 'Relative amplitude')

% Set up spectrum plot (low-frequency).
hLow = axes('Parent', f, 'OuterPosition', [0.5, 3/16, 0.5, 7/16]);
pLow = plot(hLow, freqsLow, ampsLow);
ylim(hLow, [0, 1])
title(hLow, 'Amplitude spectrum (< 1000 Hz)')
xlabel(hLow, 'Frequency (Hz)')
ylabel(hLow, 'Relative amplitude')


% Set up AudioRecorder object.
ar = audiorecorder(fs, 16, 1);

function startRecording(source, callbackdata)
    fs = 44100;
    set(startButton, 'Enable', 'off');
    set(stopButton, 'Enable', 'on');
    set(playButton, 'Enable', 'off');
    record(ar)
end

function updateSpectra()
    % Update wave plot.
    time = (1:length(y)) / fs * 1000;
    xlim(hWave, [0, max(time)])
    set(pWave, 'XData', time);
```

```
    set(pWave, 'YData', y);

    % Compute amplitude spectrum and update plot.
    NFFT = 2^nextpow2(fs);
    Y = fft(y, NFFT) / length(y);
    freqs = fs/2 * linspace(0, 1, NFFT/2 + 1) / 1000;
    amps = 2 * abs(Y(1:NFFT/2+1));
    amps = amps ./ max(amps);
    set(pSpect, 'XData', freqs);
    set(pSpect, 'YData', amps);

    % Update low-frequency section.
    freqsLow = freqs(freqs < 1) * 1000;
    ampsLow = amps(freqs < 1);
    set(pLow, 'XData', freqsLow);
    set(pLow, 'YData', ampsLow);

    % Update spectrogram.
    yS = resample(y, fsSG, fs);
    if length(yS) > fsSG * 5
        yS = yS(1:(fsSG*5));
        title(hSG, 'Spectrogram (first 5 sec)')
    else
        title(hSG, 'Spectrogram')
    end

    WINDOW = floor(fsSG/100);
    NOVERLAP = ceil(fsSG/200);
    NFFTSG = 2^nextpow2(WINDOW);
    try
        [S, F, T] = spectrogram(yS, WINDOW, NOVERLAP, NFFTSG, ...
            fsSG, 'yaxis');
        S = abs(S);
        S = S / max(max(S));
        set(hIm, 'XData', T*1000);
        set(hIm, 'YData', F/1000);
        set(hIm, 'CData', S);
        xlim(hSG, [0, max(T)*1000])
    catch
        title(hSG, 'No spectrogram - select smaller sample')
    end

end
```

```
function stopRecording(source, callbackdata)
    set(startButton, 'Enable', 'on');
    set(stopButton, 'Enable', 'off');
    set(playButton, 'Enable', 'on');
    stop(ar)
    % Extract audio.
    y = getaudiodata(ar);

    % Update.
    updateSpectra();
end

function playSample(source, callbackdata)
    sound(y, fs)
end

function openFile(source, callbackdata)
    filterSpec = {...
        '*.wav;*.flac;*.mp3;*.m4a;*.mp4;*.ogg', ...
        'All supported audio files'; ...
        '*.wav',       'WAVE files (*.wav)'; ...
        '*.flac',      'FLAC files (*.flac)'; ...
        '*.mp3',       'MPEG-3 files (*.mp3)'; ...
        '*.m4a;*.mp4', 'MPEG-4 files (*.m4a, *.mp4)'; ...
        '*.ogg',       'OGG files (*.ogg)'; ...
        '*.*',         'All files (*.*)'};
    [inFile, inPath] = uigetfile(filterSpec, 'Open audio file...');
    if any(inPath==0)
        return
    end
    inFile = fullfile(inPath, inFile);
    [y, fs] = audioread(inFile);
    y = y(:,1);
    updateSpectra();
    set(playButton, 'Enable', 'on');
end

function saveFile(source, callbackdata)
    [outFile, outPath] = uiputfile({'*.wav', 'WAVE files (*.wav)'}, ...
        'Save as...');
    if any(outPath == 0)
        return
    end
```

```
        outFile = fullfile(outPath, outFile);
        audiowrite(outFile, y, fs)
    end

    function toWorkspace(source, callbackdata)
        assignin('base', 'y', y)
        assignin('base', 'fs', fs)
        assignin('base', 'freqs', freqs * 1000)
        assignin('base', 'amps', amps)

    end

end
```

Glossary

Argument. An input to a function or operator. In the expression "2 – 1," the numbers 2 and 1 are arguments to the minus operator. In the expression "sin(θ)," the variable θ is the argument to the sine function.

ASCII. American Standard Code for Information Interchange. Common method of encoding textual data in binary. Each character takes up 7 bits, with a zero prepended to make up 1 byte.

Assignment. The process of storing a value in a variable.

Binary. A base-2 numbering system, or arithmetic based thereupon. In binary, as opposed to decimal, additional digits are needed for successive powers of two, not ten. Ubiquitous in computing. The term can also describe files that are not encoded in ASCII or some other transparent scheme.

Bit. A binary digit. A bit can take on one of two values, 0 (for "off" or false) or 1 (for "on" or true).

Byte. An ordered grouping of bits, traditionally containing eight bits. One byte can take on 255 distinct values, from `00000000` to `11111111` (`00` to `FF` in hexadecimal).

Command window. A panel in the MATLAB desktop into which commands are entered. Results from computations, as well as text output from functions, are also displayed here.

Delimited. Describing a text file whose elements are consistently separated by a prespecified character or token. Common delimiters include tabs, spaces, and commas.

Expression. A sequence of symbols or tokens that conform to the syntax of a given environment, in this case MATLAB. Expressions can include numbers, constants, string literals, variable names, function calls, mathematical operators, or other expressions.

Function. A piece of code that operates on some input and produces output, either returning it to the calling scope or creating side effects such as plots, files, or messages.

Hexadecimal. A base-16 numbering system, commonly used to compress the representation of strings of bits representing binary data. Often abbreviated as "hex."

Initialize. The process of filling up the memory allocated to a variable with an actual value. In some programming languages, declaration of variables must precede initialization. In MATLAB, variables can be declared and initialized in the same line of code.

Masking. The (often inadvertent) process of naming a variable after a built-in constant or function, which prevents further access until the variable is cleared.

Matrix. A two-dimensional array of values. In MATLAB, all elements within a matrix must be of the same type.

Objective function. A function chosen in an optimization procedure, whose minimization or maximization corresponds to the selection of the "best" or optimal parameters under the supplied definition. The decision as to whether the minimum or the maximum is sought, as well as the functional form, are determined by the scenario at hand.

Operand. One input to an operator. In the expression "5 + 3," the numbers 5 and 3 are the operands to the "+" operator.

Operator. A symbol, usually placed between two elements, that indicates some operation is to be performed on those elements (input) and its result returned as output. Common mathematical operators include addition, subtraction, multiplication, division, and exponentiation. Some operators are commutative, meaning that order is irrelevant (e.g., addition and multiplication). Other operators are sensitive to order, and yield different results when the order is changed (e.g., subtraction, division, and exponentiation).

Random access memory. A form of computer storage that (a) is volatile, meaning that its contents are erased when power is disconnected, and (b) requires the same amount of time to access any piece of information regardless of its location. Contrast with hard disks, whose access times can vary based on the file's physical location on the drive platter.

Variable. A name for a location in memory, at which data are stored. In MATLAB, variables can be of a variety of types. Variables can be included in expressions, used as operands in a mathematical formula, and passed into a function as arguments.

Workspace. A panel in the MATLAB desktop that indicates the variables that are currently assigned.

Index

Note: Page numbers in **bold** reference non-text material.

D

E

F

G

H

R

S

T